This book is gratefully dedicated to my grandmother, Fritzie, whose loving presence and shining example richly blessed my life. She taught me the importance of simplicity, self-reliance, and faith; and inspired me to discover the power of positive thinking, prayer, and holistic health. With her sparkling guidance, I learned how to live a sacred, peaceful, balanced lifestyle.

I also want to thank my guardian angels for the serendipity and the miracles that gently and lovingly guide me along my path, constantly inspiring me to celebrate life—in myself, in others, and in all living things.

"Be anxious about nothing.
Pray about everything."
— **Fritzie** (Susan's
grandmother)

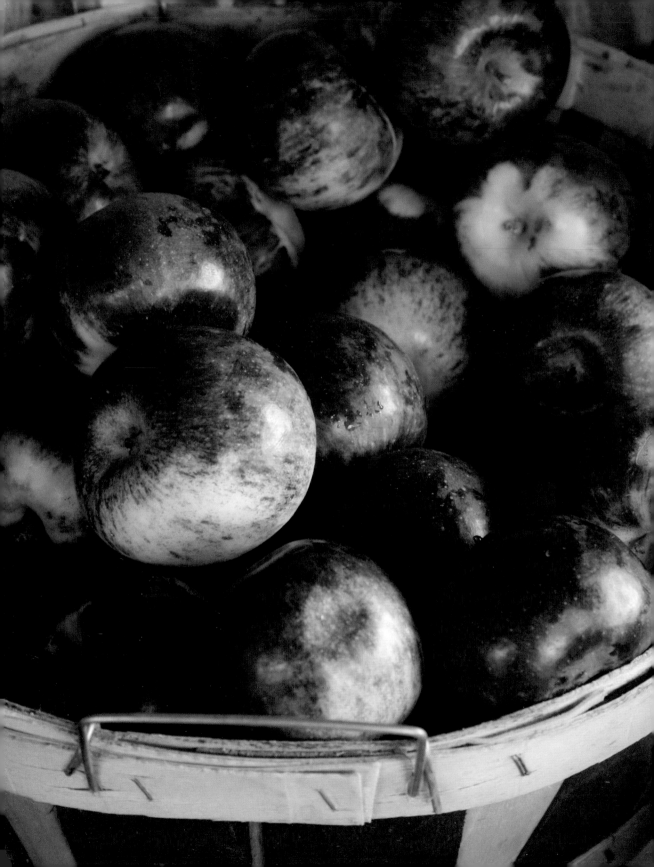

CONTENTS

PART III: Maximize Your Health

FOREWORD

by Neal Barnard, M.D.,
PRESIDENT, PHYSICIANS COMMITTEE FOR RESPONSIBLE MEDICINE

This book is more than a collection of great recipes. It's a road to health. You certainly will find wonderful recipes here, and each one is healthful and simple to prepare. Many of these lovely meals will feel like old friends. Many others will entice you to try new tastes. You'll love their scent and flavor, and how good you feel when you make them part of your life.

But this book is more than that. It's a pathway that leads from wherever you find yourself at the moment to the best health you can imagine.

When I first learned about Susan Smith Jones and her gift for guiding people to health, I could see that she knew what she was talking about. Don't let her warmth and gentle writing style fool you. The prescription she offers has been proven by clinical research studies. Her books are potentially the most powerful, life-changing guides you'll ever hold in your hands.

For many years, my research team has tested how diet changes can tackle difficult health problems. Their power is truly surprising. They boost your energy, make you feel and look younger, and trim away unwanted pounds. If you have a more serious health challenge, simple diet changes can help you, too. Research shows that they can tackle arthritis, cholesterol problems, high blood pressure, hormone imbalances, cancer, digestive problems, headaches, and many other health concerns.

Beginning in 2003, the National Institutes of Health supported our research on diet and diabetes. As our research participants began their nutritional changes, their bodies started to transform. Pounds began to melt away. Cholesterol levels plummeted. And day after day, my phone rang with participants telling me that their blood sugars were finally returning toward normal. One after another was able to reduce—or even eliminate—the medications they'd taken, in some cases, for years.

When you've discovered a way to profoundly change your life, you never look back. At the beginning, you might have been a bit unsure. But now that you know how good you can feel, you want to keep going. Your tastes and your body have forever changed. That's what is in store for you as you let this esteemed author, culinary instructor, advice columnist, and motivational speaker, Susan Smith Jones, guide you to vibrant health and youthful vitality.

If you're already familiar with Susan's work, jump in. You won't be disappointed. If her approach is new to you, let me encourage you to carefully read her nutritional recommendations, and then page through the recipes and simply try them out. See which ones call to you the most. And then when you're ready, take a three-week period and make every meal fit her recommended guidelines. By the end of the trial, you'll be surprised by how good you feel, and your tastes will have transformed, too. You'll find that healthful foods attract you like never before, and old and unhealthy foods are soon forgotten.

Let me also encourage you to heed Susan's advice for other parts of your life, too. When she encourages you to get a good night's sleep, this is vitally important advice. Sleep is when you reset your appetite control and pain control. It's when your energy regroups for the day to come. Physical activity, nurturing relationships, and a sense of purpose are part of a healthy life, too, and Susan has brought all of these to the fore, as well.

I wish you the best in exploring these healthful and delicious foods, and I hope you'll feel as rewarded as I have.

(Neal's Website: **www.nutritionmd.org**)

FOREWORD

by Victoria Moran,
THE AUTHOR OF *CREATING A CHARMED LIFE* AND *FIT FROM WITHIN*

There's good health and poor health. Most people have some degree of one or the other. But there is another category, rare and wonderful: *health bliss.* And one more person stands to experience it: you, as you put into practice what you'll learn in this book.

Leave it to Susan Smith Jones to apply the word *bliss,* a state she knows so well, to the health of body and mind. I've observed this amazing woman for more than 25 years (I know—she looks as if she were in kindergarten 25 years ago—that alone is proof that this way of life works). In all this time, I've known her to walk her talk without a misstep. After a serious automobile accident that caused doctors to say she'd barely walk again, Susan put into practice the way of eating and living detailed in this book, as well as the spiritual tools of affirmation, meditation, and faith-filled prayer. As a result, she walked . . . and ran . . . and bungee jumped, parachuted, kayaked, competed in triathlons, and hiked mountains. She still does. It's no wonder that the President's Council on Physical Fitness and Sports selected Susan as one of ten Healthy American Fitness Leaders.

This is health bliss. It's more than freedom from disease or simply having enough energy to get through the day. It's a true state of bliss—defined as "ecstasy," "rapture," and "perfect happiness." This is what everyone wants and what this readable and content-packed book offers us all.

Susan started us on this road with her two previous best-selling Hay House books in this illustrious three-book healthy-living series: *The Healing Power of NatureFoods* and *Health Bliss: 50 Revitalizing NatureFoods & Lifestyle Choices to Promote Vibrant Health*. I highly recommend these books as companion guides or a gift set for your family and friends, yet you can jump into *Recipes for Health Bliss* with no prerequisites. The recipes Susan creates and shares here are a veritable "food pharmacy" of fresh, natural, delicious dishes that will start you on your way to a blissfully vibrant life. You'll love these recipes that allow you to interact with beautiful, colorful foods straight from nature. If you're not a cook and find the culinary arts a bit intimidating, rest assured that the dishes are simple, quick, and use ingredients easily found at your farmers market, natural-food store, or any large supermarket.

Be sure as you indulge in *Recipes for Health Bliss* that you read between the lines—or in this case, between the recipes. This isn't just a cookbook (or largely "cookless book" since many of the recipes classify as "living foods"). It's also a guide to dietary, attitudinal, and lifestyle changes that guarantee you high-level health and a more fulfilling life. You can make these transitions gradually—a wonderful green smoothie today, a scrumptious glass of fresh vegetable juice tomorrow—and feel the changes taking place in your body and mind one day at a time.

As you apply Susan's suggestions in your kitchen and life, you'll be embarking on a great adventure in both self-care and compassion. These recipes are plant based and body friendly, meaning that you can easily process the food and extract the nutrients. The result is a younger, more attractive, more vital you—*and* no animal has to suffer or die for your dinner. This lifts a burden from your digestive system and from your soul, because each of us is, after all, a tiny, brilliant part of the One Life expressing in myriad forms.

These pages hold a powerful message, as well as a plethora of fabulous recipes, and the messenger is the real deal. Read with an open mind and a ready blender. Great things are about to happen for your body and in your life.

(Victoria's Website: **www.victoriamoran.com**)

"When you put your force and energy behind something, the results will be powerful."

— Alexandra Stoddard

INTRODUCTION

"Each patient carries his own doctor inside him."

— ALBERT SCHWEITZER

One of the main reasons I wrote this book is because I like to make people feel good—the kind of good that comes from an unexpected, deep belly laugh and enjoying nutritious, delectable food—food that also just happens to help heal the body. It's similar to the way your favorite childhood memory gives you a tingle and puts a smile on your face whenever it comes to you, even as you rush through an activity-filled day in a busy city or community far away from where you grew up.

My love for food and creating recipes started when I was a little girl and I watched my mom and grandmother spending lots of time in the kitchen, creating meals that brought all of us kids and our playmates out of our rooms or in from the yard. Even during holidays, my mom would always create extra room at our table for friends who were far away from their relatives or who didn't have any family. We also invited a few service members from nearby military bases who were far away from their homes. These were good times, and great food was always the hub of the wheel, which incited lots of laughter, enjoyable conversations, and countless "Yums."

Even to this day, I've adopted my mom's and grandmother's passion for sharing good food, as my neighbors, friends, and family can attest. I'm always making gifts of homemade creations to help brighten their days in some small way. It's one of my greatest passions in life: creating wonderful dishes and sharing my love for food and healthy living with as many people as possible. My hope is that this book will inspire you to create your own healthy meals; share them with family and friends; and find other simple ways to adopt a more nurturing lifestyle as I describe in these pages.

It's a thrill for me to have this opportunity to share my recipes with you. They're an outgrowth of decades of research and experimentation in the field of healthful living. As a young woman, I had a dream that someday I'd discover the secrets of a long life of fitness, vibrant health, youthful vigor, and exquisite joy. I'm happy to say that my dream came true, and I'm grateful to be able to share my experiences with you.

As you read this book, I hope you feel as though we're sitting across from each other at the kitchen table, visiting and chatting as friends. I already know that we have some things in common since you've chosen to read a book filled with nutritious recipes and health tips. I'm eager to share with you the secrets that have led to success for thousands of people, and I know that they can do the same for *you!*

True Health and Wholeness

If you've read any of my other books, then you're aware that my approach to creating vibrant health is holistic. If you're new to my work, here's a brief overview of my perspective and philosophy:

Health is our normal state of being, and it comes about as a result of living in harmony with nature. Lasting wellness can be achieved and maintained only through healthful living in all of its aspects. You see, health is more than the absence of disease; it refers to a vibrant quality of life. An intricate relationship links the brain, the hormone system, and the immune system, which means that feeling good is a physical, mental, and emotional experience.

Being radiantly healthy involves recognizing that all aspects of life are interrelated and must be integrated if you're to realize your full potential. In our increasingly complicated society, to become well—and *stay* that way—takes awareness and a commitment to meeting the needs of your body, mind, and spirit.

The body reflects the mind and emotions, and the mind and emotions reflect the spirit. For example, when the physical self is in good shape—fit, toned, and strong—the mind is affected positively, resulting in high self-esteem and self-confidence. The opposite is also true. The out-of-shape, sluggish, and weak body has a negative effect on mental function, which contributes to lowered self-esteem and a negative outlook on life.

The importance of health to satisfaction and success in life has always been known. As early as 300 B.C., Herophilus wrote: "When health is absent, wisdom cannot reveal itself, art cannot become manifest, strength cannot be exerted, wealth is useless, and reason is powerless." In a recent Gallup survey, 75 percent of respondents rated optimism, clean environment, stress control, good relationships, and satisfying work as very important contributors to health. People who enjoy what they do and who feel a sense of control over their lives tend to be healthier.

Eating right, exercising regularly, thinking positively, and keeping stress levels down can do more than add a few years to your life span. They can improve the *quality* of your life, especially in later years. And Americans are living longer than ever before; the average life span for women is now around 87 years.

Full-Spectrum Health

A healthful diet is extremely important, and it's virtually impossible to enjoy the highest levels of health without it. But good food alone can't ensure radiant health or youthful vitality. Extensive research in the field of health and wellness over the past 35 years indicates that there are at least 20 essential factors that must be integrated and balanced in your life if vibrancy is what you want. These include fresh air and sunshine, plenty of rest and sleep, avoidance of addictions, exercise, wholesome nutrition, deep breathing, a clean body, a balanced life, systematic *undereating,* a deep respect for life, high self-esteem, daily respites of solitude and silence, a positive attitude, and a sense of belonging. In my three-book Hay House series, *The Healing Power of NatureFoods; Health Bliss;* and this book, *Recipes for Health Bliss,* I've touched on all of these topics, some in great depth.

Eating for Health

In this third book of the series, I'll focus on the best foods and recipes to enhance your health and life. For the past 25 years, I've been a culinary instructor and have worked with groups, families, and individuals, teaching them how to select excellent foods and how to prepare healthful meals that everyone will love. One of my passions has been to teach my clients how to make the simple dietary changes that result in the most profound difference in health and vitality. As an example, I share a story in Chapter 1 about one of my clients, Danielle, whom I wrote about in *Health Bliss.* I include her journey in case you haven't read that book yet. The dietary and lifestyle changes that her family undertook will inspire you to make positive shifts in your life, too.

Additionally, you'll find a variety of recipes for all occasions within these pages. You'll also learn about my favorite kitchen gadgets, which can help save you a lot of preparation time. Let's face it—very few of us have hours each day to spend in the kitchen making complicated meals. My goal is to provide you with easy-to-prepare recipes and a wide range of food tips, but I won't stop there. I'll also present additional health recommendations designed to help you live a vibrantly healthy life—physically, mentally, emotionally, and spiritually.

Embrace Patience

As you change your diet from one that encourages sickness and fatigue to one that produces optimal wellness, don't be surprised if you feel a tad worse before you begin to feel better. An initial negative change is often a sign that your body is housecleaning, that it's trying to heal itself. Most unhealthful foods are highly concentrated and habit forming (yes, just like drugs), so it should come as no surprise that you may need to go through a short period of withdrawal. Don't let this temporary discomfort dissuade you from making the switch. Persist. The rich rewards will come sooner than you think. Supply your body only with what it needs, and it will take care of the rest.

It boils down to this: *How much do you want to celebrate life and experience vibrancy?* It's up to you. Choose today to be in alignment with nature's laws of health and healing. Persistence and commitment are the keys. How you care for your body reveals your inner sense of self-worth. Nurturing yourself with fresh foods, pure water, clean air, sunshine, rest, and exercise will lead you to the level of radiant health you've always dreamed of having. I encourage you to get copies of the first two books in this healthy-living series so that you have at your fingertips all of the tools and information necessary to create your very best life.

I salute your great adventure and hope to meet you someday, somewhere along the way.

"If we did all the things we are capable of doing,
we would literally astound ourselves."

— THOMAS ALVA EDISON

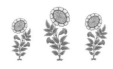

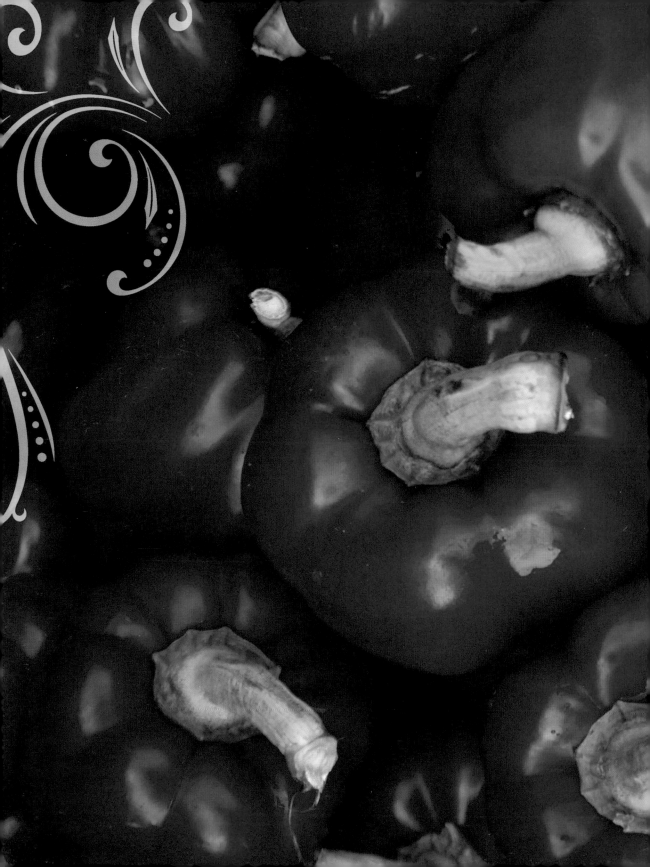

PART I

RETHINK YOUR DIET

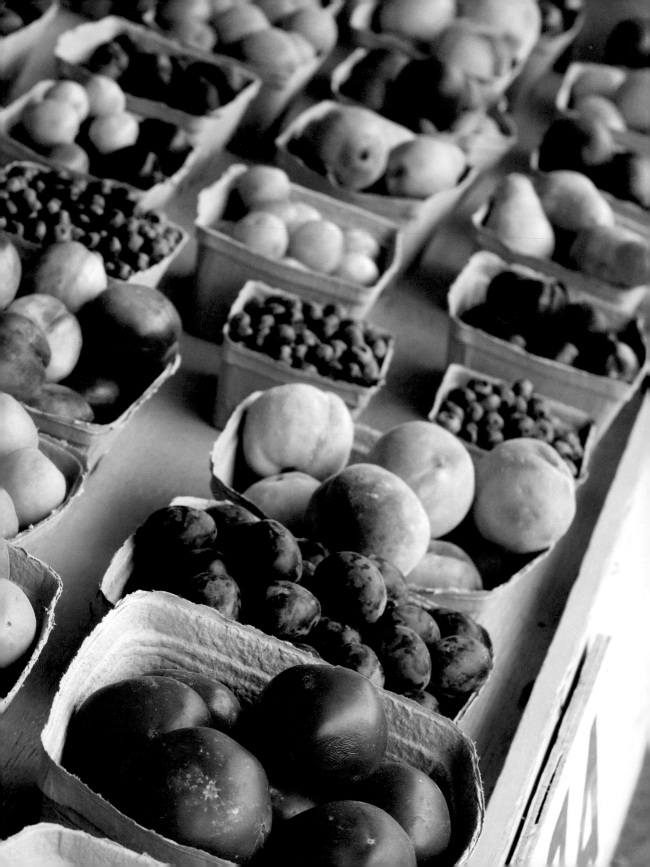

CHAPTER 1

QUANTUM NUTRITION

"Nothing will benefit human health and increase the chances for survival of life on earth as much as the evolution to a vegetarian diet."

— ALBERT EINSTEIN

Last year, the president of a major American corporation—a very wealthy 55-year-old whom I'll call Arthur—came to me for a consultation. Arthur wasn't warm and fuzzy. He was impatient, aggressive (sometimes hostile), and totally unaware of how to maintain his well-being. Each week, he routinely put in six or seven long, pressure-packed days at the office or traveling. He always had to be first, always had to be right, and always had to be busy with work to feel worthwhile. Playful behavior was not part of his lifestyle. A fancier of rich meals, he ate vast quantities of cheese, ice cream, steak, butter, processed foods, and cream sauces. He knew his diet was loaded with cholesterol and fat, but he loved it all the same. As he once told me (paraphrasing Oscar Wilde), when it came to food, he could resist anything but temptation. The most vigorous exercise he got was shifting the gears of one of his expensive sports cars.

Arthur was chronically stressed and fatigued, but he thought that his hot tub and a drink were all he needed to relax. It wasn't until he began to sink into a deep depression that his wife urged him to get a medical checkup, his first in more than five years. The results came as a shock. Arthur learned that he had high blood pressure and serious hardening of the arteries. The cardiologist advised him to undergo quadruple-bypass surgery and warned him that if he didn't make some changes in his way of life immediately, he was headed for a heart attack within six months.

As providence would have it, the following day a friend of Arthur's, having heard about the prognosis, recommended that he follow the holistic-health and stress-reduction regimens I write about in my books. So Arthur sought me out and asked me to help him develop a wellness program. I'd never worked with anyone who was quite so desperate and who led such an unhealthy life, but I promised that I'd try to help him.

Arthur's experiences and adventures over the months since then have been a great inspiration to me. During our first visit, he made an important choice— he chose to make a commitment to change his life and to be healthy. Today, he and his entire family are the picture of health. Recently, they participated together in a 10K run, and the following day they left for a two-week health-and-fitness vacation. You can follow suit.

Simple Lifestyle Changes Make the Biggest Difference

I can't overemphasize the importance of making a commitment to small improvements in day-to-day food choices and the need to reprogram and retrain your senses to release self-limiting beliefs and habits. I touched on these commitments in my book *Health Bliss;* if you haven't read it yet, what follows is a brief recap:

Your primary goal on this quantum-nutrition program is to get to the point where you're eating an abundance of the highest-quality foods—especially leafy-green vegetables—with as many raw, living items as possible. Almost 2,500 years ago, Pythagoras said, "Choose what is best; habit will soon render it agreeable and easy." His sagacious words are just as relevant today as they were back then, especially when it comes to establishing new healthful food and lifestyle customs.

After decades of poor choices, you probably harbor some negative programming about your eating habits, which can undermine your best intentions if you aren't careful. It almost always leads you to seek immediate gratification rather than long-term satisfaction. Your emotionally entrenched habits don't care if you achieve your goal of a fit, lean, healthy body. Driven by only these impulses, you want to feel good right now. At times like these, you need to rely on your sober, rational mind (not the *rationalizing* mind that's all too willing to go along with the emotionally driven idea that you need a candy bar or a cupcake).

You must learn to detach from your negative programming and bad habits in order to achieve your long-term goals. Whether regarding food or something else, the difficulty in resisting sensory desire comes from the force of conditioning. Every time you receive negative reinforcement, you lose a little of your freedom and your capacity to choose. To begin your transformation, start becoming aware of what you're consuming. If you're only eating at the table, at mealtimes, and when you're hungry, you can more easily focus on your food. When your attention is divided, you're more likely to snack compulsively rather than from hunger. Automatic eating occurs frequently in front of the television or at the movie theater, parties, or sporting events. Try to avoid consuming anything in these settings, or make a point to have healthful foods available.

The entire process of eating needs to be given your full attention for you to get the maximum benefits. Be conscious of the hunger you feel and how the food looks and smells as you prepare it, serve it, and eat it. Become aware of the table setting's appearance. How does the food taste? Be conscious of its texture, your chewing, your breathing, and how you feel while you're eating. Finally, notice and be grateful for the feelings of lightness and high energy derived from the meal. By embracing this attitude, you can begin to appreciate simple, wholesome foods and to eat less, while still feeling completely satisfied.

Stop eating just before you feel really full. By doing so, you begin reprogramming your subconscious and cease letting your habits control you. Stopping short of satiety helps you savor your food and allows you to be free and in charge of your choices. Likewise, begin eliminating those things that you know are harmful. Retrain your senses to seek out and prefer only those ingredients that meet your body's needs. I find that meditating for a few minutes before each meal is a powerful tool that fosters good choices and promotes health and harmony.

Your taste buds will quickly change and adapt to your new, healthful diet. For example, the whole-grain bread that initially seemed heavy and grainy will soon taste chewy and flavorful. Feeling better and looking marvelous will quickly compensate for the loss of dubious thrills of the past, such as fried chicken, white bread, ice cream, candy, and potato chips. You'll find yourself looking forward to more healthful pleasures, such as the taste of ripe papaya; luscious strawberries; blueberries; pineapple; sweet, juicy grapes; a crisp garden salad; brown rice or quinoa with steamed vegetables; and sweet potatoes smothered in sautéed onions, broccoli, and mushrooms.

Danielle's Story: Change Your Diet, Change Your Life

Danielle is a great example of how changing your diet and adding more living, whole foods can not only assist with weight loss, but also improve every aspect of your family life and self-esteem. Married with three children—ages five, eight, and eleven—Danielle initially came to me for motivation and help in losing some fat, toning up her body, and increasing her energy. As a first step, I asked her to keep a seven-day food diary and record exactly what and when she ate. Like all of my new clients, she was instructed not to eat differently simply because I'd be looking at the list; she had to be honest and write everything down, because there's no other way to make a true evaluation.

When I received her food diary, it was quite apparent why she'd gained almost 30 pounds in a year and why she always felt enervated. Her diet was about 60 percent fat, almost all of the carbohydrates she consumed were refined, she usually skipped breakfast because she was too busy getting the kids ready for school, and she always ate late at night. Her diary looked like an encyclopedia of deleterious eating habits! She rarely included raw foods in the family diet, explaining that it took too long to chew them. Her kids also disliked uncooked ingredients, so she rarely had fruits or salad vegetables in the house.

As I inquired more about her family life, routines, and eating habits, I learned that all of her children were on the heavy side. The oldest girl was starting to be ridiculed in school because of her size. Not surprisingly, Danielle told me that her husband also needed to lose about 40 pounds. His blood pressure, cholesterol, and triglycerides were much too high, and his doctor had suggested that he go on a diet.

My initial evaluation of how this family ate and lived led me to suggest something out of the ordinary. Knowing that they had a large house with a guest room next to the kitchen, I asked if I could stay with them from Thursday through Saturday night. I wanted to experience their lifestyle as a family, to see how they lived at home, when and what they ate, and how they spent their time when they weren't eating, in order to coach them toward a healthier path. Yes, I brought most of my own food, and I simply observed like a butterfly on the wall and took lots of notes. I had Danielle's permission to look through the pantry and refrigerator and all of the kitchen cupboards when they were out of the house. Sure enough, there were almost no fresh, whole foods.

At mealtime, everyone salted the dishes before tasting them; and their dining table was never without canned sodas or processed fruit juices, butter, sour cream, and mounds of cheese. All five of them consumed their meals quickly, without much conversation and without putting the utensils down between bites. I think most of their overeating was unintentional, since they had no idea that many popular foods contain hidden sugar and oils that are put there to stimulate the taste buds.

This family needed a complete health makeover. With Danielle's consent, I made a clean sweep of her kitchen. The rest of her family agreed to go along with this "experiment," although they were far from enthusiastic. I removed all refined carbohydrates, including pasta, white rice, low-fiber cereals, pancake and cookie mixes, white breads, and bagels . . . and replaced these with high-fiber breads and whole grains. I also rid their kitchen of margarine, mayonnaise, vegetable shortenings, and oils. Next, I took away all of the milk and cheese products. Those high-fat, calorie-loaded cheese slices provide between 80 and 140 calories per one-ounce slice, depending on the fat content. I replaced the cow's milk with raw-nut and seed milks. After about two weeks of adapting to the new tastes, it turned out that they all loved the vanilla-flavored almond beverage the best.

I took the entire family to the nearest health-food store and showed them all of the nutritious alternatives, such as veggie burgers and whole-grain pastas, and then I led them to the produce section. They were enthralled by all of the colors and varieties of fruits and vegetables, many of which they'd never seen before. We purchased some of the most familiar—organic apples, oranges, pears, grapes, bananas, and strawberries.

In place of sodas and other canned drinks, I taught them how to make their own juice. The kids loved juicing and actually wanted to take it over as their daily job. Of course, I also encouraged them to start drinking more water. Danielle's husband confessed to me secretly that he couldn't remember having more than about six glasses of water per week. When I told him how much purified, alkalinized water I drink every day, he almost collapsed in shock. I use the following formula: start with your body weight in pounds (say 120 pounds), divide it in half (60 pounds), and drink the same number (60) of ounces of water each day. If you weigh more than 200 pounds, strive for at least eight glasses (eight ounces each) of water daily.

It took about one month for the family to adjust their taste buds to the new flavors, textures, and colors. They basically switched from a white and beige diet to a banquet of rainbow colors. I introduced them to the benefits of consuming raw foods and showed them several simple recipes that they could enjoy often. They were eager to move in this new direction. After several "uncooking" lessons, Danielle found that it wasn't so hard to prepare healthier meals. Almost half of the family's diet became raw foods, with an abundance of fresh fruits and vegetables. When you fill up on these things, you nourish your body and actually lose much of your desire for processed foods.

After three months, as a result of eating more fiber and more nutritious ingredients, the family members all lost weight, had more energy and balanced moods, and enjoyed a greater sense of well-being that resulted in more positive attitudes all around. I encouraged them all to be more active instead of hanging out in front of televisions or computers most nights and weekends, and their higher activity resulted in sounder sleep for everyone. Danielle's oldest daughter lost weight and joined an after-school sports team, which ended the ridicule and helped her self-esteem soar.

It's truly remarkable how making a few basic changes in your diet can profoundly affect every area of your life. The one shift that this family found most difficult was my suggestion to pick one day each week to only eat raw food. I suggested that they not select a weekend day, but rather a Tuesday, Wednesday, or Thursday. They chose Thursday, and from morning through evening ate only living foods—lots of fruits and vegetables, salads, and a variety of other fun things, including nut butters, sprouts, sauces, and soups—even cookies and other desserts. The family came to appreciate Danielle's gift for experimenting with, and creating, new raw meals. A few weeks into their new health regimen, they started having friends over for meals to sample their delicious "health-nut food"!

Since you're reading this book, I'm confident that it's time for *you* to make some changes in your diet. Even though you may not be eager to overhaul your entire food program, at least begin by adding more and more of the recipes into your diet. You might start by eating healthful breakfasts each day, or eating only nutritious dishes on two or more days per week. This gentle approach will assist you in bringing more beneficial foods into your diet by spacing them out over the week. You'll feel lighter and more energetic immediately, simply from taking this small step.

Sleepless in America

In addition to making a clean sweep of Danielle's kitchen, restocking it with better food choices, and supporting the family in being more physically active, I also encouraged everyone to make sleep a top priority—a nonnegotiable, regular habit. Lack of sleep undermines your body's ability to deal with stress and maintain a healthy weight. One way to tell if you're getting enough shut-eye is to see if you wake at a regular time without an alarm. If you require a buzzer to get out of bed in the morning, you're not getting enough rest.

How much sleep do you really need each day? Adults require eight and a quarter hours of sleep nightly to maximize their ability to function daily. Adolescents need 9 and a quarter hours; preschoolers should get 12 hours; toddlers need 13 hours; and babies require 14 to 18 hours of sleep every day.

Researchers are discovering that sleep affects the hormones that regulate satiety, hunger, and how efficiently you burn calories. Put simply, too little sleep makes you hungry, especially for things that are high in calories and low in nutritional value. These include processed junk foods, especially those made with white sugar and flour, and fried foods such as French fries and potato chips. Moreover, lack of sleep also primes your body to hold on to the calories you eat.

Are you interested in slimming down? If so, this may provide some help: At Columbia University in New York City, researchers found that people who slept six hours a night were 23 percent more likely to be obese than people who slept between seven and nine hours. Those who snoozed for five hours were 50 percent more likely—while those who slept four hours or less were 73 percent more likely—to be obese. So if you're eager to drop a few pounds, make getting ample sleep each night a nonnegotiable habit in your lifestyle.

In my private practice as well as in my holistic-health seminars around the country, I also recommend quality sleep because it makes for better relationships. If everyone would just get more rest, people would be more thoughtful toward one another, and family dynamics would run more smoothly. We'd all be happier and be in better moods—adults and children alike. What a wonderful gift that would be to give to our family, friends, and business associates. Think of how much our communities would benefit. (Please refer to my book *Health Bliss* to read more about the importance of sleep.)

Dairy-Free Recipes

If you have allergies, you'll be happy to know that all of the recipes in this book are dairy free. For health and ethical reasons, I choose not to eat any dairy products; and with only a very few rare, unavoidable exceptions, I haven't eaten them for years. When I announce this at my workshops, people inevitably ask what I use in place of milk. Excellent substitutes include numerous nut milks, oat milk, rice milk, hemp milk, and soy milk. All of these are available in natural-food stores and come in plain, vanilla, chocolate, low-fat, nonfat, and organic. I always purchase organic whenever possible.

In Chapter 2, I've included a recipe for making your own nut milks (and there are even more, as well as recipes for nut cheeses, in my book BE HEALTHY~STAY BALANCED). You also can make or purchase soy yogurt, soy cheese, soy cream cheese, and soy sour cream, so you won't miss your dairy. Soy may have a special health benefit since it contains phytoestrogens. Numerous studies have confirmed that women who eat foods rich in these compounds seem to have fewer symptoms of PMS and menopause.

I don't have the space here to describe all of the reasons why researchers have become so concerned about dairy products. The list is simply too long. Suffice it to say, even if you choose to include dairy in your diet, I suggest that you limit it to very small portions once or twice per week. I will, however, describe just a few of the problems associated with this category of food.

Milk is the leading cause of iron-deficiency anemia in children. Milk allergies are very common in kids and can cause sinus problems, diarrhea, constipation, and fatigue. These allergies are the leading cause of the chronic ear infections that plague up to 40 percent of all children under the age of six, and they're also linked to behavior problems and the disturbing rise in childhood asthma. Such allergies are equally common in adults and produce similar symptoms. Milk is touted as "nature's perfect food," but most African Americans (70 percent), Asian

Americans (95 percent), Native Americans (74 percent), and Hispanic Americans (53 percent) are lactose intolerant.

Dairy products have no dietary fiber. Among other problems, diets low in fiber contribute to constipation and other related diseases (varicose veins, hemorrhoids, and hiatal hernia). There's evidence that immune-system reactions to dairy proteins may cause and/or aggravate rheumatoid arthritis in some people, and there are clear links between dairy products and osteoporosis, obesity, cancer, allergies, and diabetes. High-fat dairy products, such as whole milk and cheese, are significant contributors to high cholesterol levels and heart disease, and low-fat or fat-free versions may be culprits as well. Worldwide, the incidence of type 1 diabetes correlates to the amount of dairy products consumed; so does breast cancer.

Symptoms associated with consumption of dietary estrogen from dairy and meat products include acceleration of the aging process; decreased sex drive; depression; fatigue; irritability; decreased metabolism; water retention and bloating; and fat gain, especially around the abdomen, hips, and thighs—just to name a few.

Most of the clients who come to me have at least some weight issues and want to reduce fat. Those who eliminate dairy have a much easier time losing weight than those who don't. Most even say that the weight came off easily and effortlessly when they gave up dairy as well as all other animal products.

Don't take chances with your health! The risks associated with milk and dairy products are well documented. If these products still play a role in your diet, start cutting back. Check at your natural-food store for more healthful substitutes.

Rejuvenating Your Taste Buds

Throughout the recipe sections, you'll see references to Bragg Liquid Amino Acids, low-sodium tamari, shoyu, oil, sea salt, and various soy products. I include these because I want to help ease your transition from the standard American diet (SAD) to a healthier way of eating. As your taste buds acclimate to the heavenly, unseasoned flavors of whole natural foods, you can eliminate most of these ingredients or replace them with more healthful substitutes. Excess consumption of sodium, extracted oils, and processed foods (organic or not) carry health risks; and so does anything made with aspartame. All you need to do is search the Internet and you'll discover why it's such a poison to the body. I'll never eat anything to which aspartame has been added. So as you get more experienced, keep these products to a minimum. When I use salt, I use Celtic Sea Salt (available in natural-food stores, or check the Resources section of this book).

Let's Get Started

Now it's time to begin making the most healthful and delicious recipes I know. And since nothing tastes quite as refreshing as a delicious, thirst-quenching drink, let's start with juices and smoothies. After that, you'll find a cornucopia of delights for every occasion!

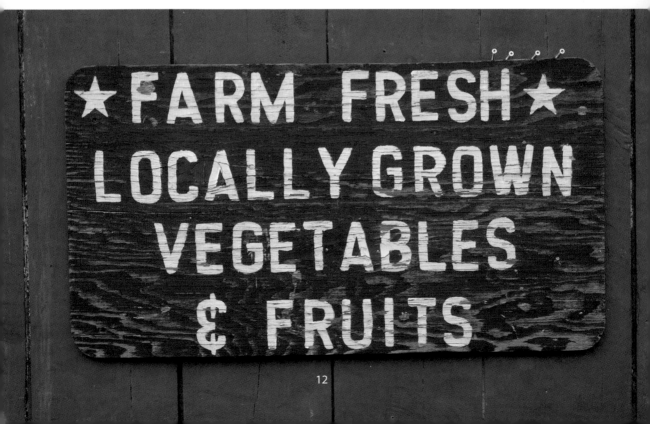

CHAPTER 2

JUICES & SMOOTHIES

*"I look younger. My skin is more supple now, and
I have fewer wrinkles than I did before eating raw food."*

— CAROL ALT, SUPERMODEL

Juicing is one of the easiest, most efficient, and delicious ways to ensure that you're meeting your daily produce quota—I recommend 7 to 12 servings daily. Most people think of fresh juices and smoothies as snacks, but they can be meals in themselves, especially when you don't have much time. While I don't advise eating on the run—it's terrible for the digestion—we all have to do it sometimes. But just because you need to grab something quick doesn't mean you need to make a poor choice. I've been drinking fresh juices for more than 35 years. In fact, I make a habit of doing a one-day "juice fast" (drinking only fresh, wholesome, organic juices) each week to give my digestive system a rest. I always wake up the next day feeling lighter, more energetic, and more positive.

When shopping for fresh fruits and vegetables for juicing, buy organic whenever possible and always choose the freshest varieties available. If you can't buy organic, make sure to wash your produce well. Even if you get produce without pesticides, you'll still want to be sure to rinse everything thoroughly. There are many commercial produce washes available, but I like to make my own. Here's my recipe: Fill your sink with cold water, and add four tablespoons of salt and the juice of a lemon. Soak fruits and vegetables for ten minutes, then rinse under cold water. You also can substitute ¼ cup white vinegar for the lemon.

After your produce is washed, all you need to do is cut it into pieces to fit the size of your juicer or blender, and you're ready to roll. I'm a big fan of both the Champion Juicer and The Total Blender. (See the Resources section for ordering information.)

Before I drink fresh juices, whether fruit or vegetable based, I usually drink a glass of water first. Doing this helps dilute the concentrated fruit sugars while allowing me to enjoy my juice full strength, which means I get the full flavor. It also fills me up a bit, which discourages "overdrinking." Make sure you sip slowly and don't gulp. Try using beautiful goblets and glasses that you can pre-chill in the freezer. The cold glass helps keep the juice cool and adds a touch of simple elegance.

Now let's go into the kitchen and prepare some of the most healthful recipes imaginable. I know you'll enjoy these juices and smoothies as much as I do.

WEIGHT-LOSS EXPRESS

This easy-to-prepare, delicious juice supercharges metabolism and supplies an abundance of synergistically balanced nutrients that the cells can use immediately to energize your body. If you like carrot juice, you'll love this weight-loss special.

Serves 1–2.

1 medium apple, peeled and quartered
2 large or 3 medium carrots, cut to juicer size
2 stalks celery
3-inch piece of cucumber, peeled and halved
½ cup parsley leaves and stems
½ small lemon (with peel, if organic)
¼- to 2-inch piece of fresh ginger (depending on how
    "gingery" you want it; I use a 2-inch piece)
1–2 Tbsp. protein powder

Juice all produce ingredients, blend in the powder, and serve.

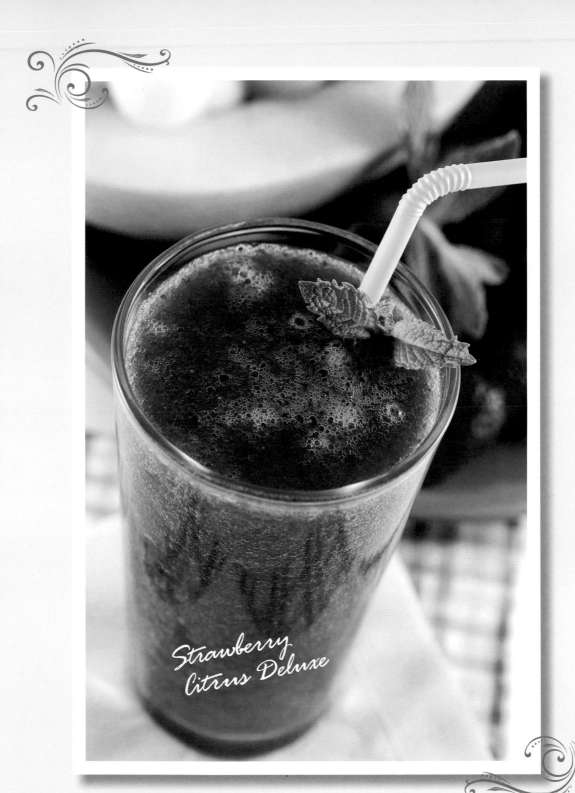

Strawberry
Citrus Deluxe

STRAWBERRY CITRUS DELUXE

This fruit-juice blend is as delicious as it is beautiful. Enjoy it at any time of the day.

Serves 1–2.

1 ruby red grapefruit, peeled and quartered (leaving pithy part on is okay)
2 tangerines, peeled and halved
1 orange, peeled and quartered
6 large strawberries, green tops included
¼-inch piece of fresh ginger (optional)

Juice all ingredients and serve.

FYI: Strawberries

Strawberries are a good source of vitamins A and C, beta-carotene, folic acid, and potassium. They're also anticancer, antiviral, and antibacterial.

TOP OF THE MORNING

If you don't have much time for breakfast but want a healthy start to your day, this vegetable and fruit combination fits the bill. I've enjoyed this drink several times each week for three decades.

Serves 1–2.

3 medium carrots
1 apple
1 large stalk celery
1 stalk broccoli, with florets
⅓ cup parsley
¼ sweet bell pepper (red, yellow, or orange)
½ small beet
¼ lemon wedge (with peel, if organic)
¼-inch piece of ginger

Juice all ingredients and serve.

CALCIUM COOLER

This juice is bright green and has a super-fresh taste. It's a great source of calcium and is loaded with the antioxidant power of the leafy greens.
Serves 1–2.

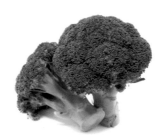

3 organic green apples
2 medium kale leaves
1 stalk broccoli with florets
4 large leaves spinach, washed well
3 sprigs fresh mint
¼ lemon wedge (with peel, if organic)

Juice all ingredients and serve.

FYI: Apples

Apples are a super health food. They help relieve constipation, reactivate beneficial gut bacteria, reduce total cholesterol, and assist in detoxifying the body.

CAROTENE COCKTAIL

Do you want to revitalize your skin and supercharge your energy? If so, this is the juice for you.
Serves 2.

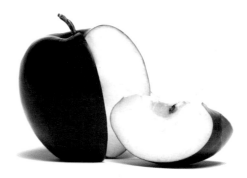

3 medium carrots
1 large red apple
1 large ripe tomato, quartered
½ sweet bell pepper (red, yellow, or orange)
½ cup baby spinach
¼ cup parsley
¼ wedge lemon (with peel, if organic)
¼-inch piece of fresh ginger

Juice all ingredients and serve.

FYI: Ginger

Ginger has a long and honored tradition in folk medicine. Some of its benefits include preventing motion sickness, quelling nausea and morning sickness, reducing inflammation, and relieving menstrual cramps. It's also great for improving circulation, which is one of the reasons I add it to many of my juices. To help relieve the chills and congestion of a cold, you can make ginger tea by simmering one or two slices of fresh ginger root in a few cups of water for 10 minutes. I like to add a pinch of cinnamon and a few drops of fresh lemon juice for piquancy.

TROPICAL-FRUIT COCKTAIL

This colorful juice helps reduce inflammation, in addition to providing vitamin C, calcium, magnesium, and potassium.

Serves 1–2.

2 cups pineapple, peeled
1 ruby red grapefruit, peeled (leaving pithy part on is okay)
2 firm kiwis, peeled
4 strawberries, green tops included

Juice all ingredients and serve.

FYI: Pineapple & Grapefruit

Pineapple contains bromelain, a potent digestive enzyme that scavenges bacteria and parasites. Ruby red grapefruit has more beta-carotene than the pink or white varieties. Putting a bit of essential oil of grapefruit (you can find it at your natural-food store) on the inside of your wrist will help keep your appetite at bay and preclude overeating. This oil isn't for internal use—rather it's intended to be used on your skin. It's one of my fragrances of choice, and I often use it as my signature scent.

BERRY-CHERRY ZING

Believe me, it's worth the time it takes to pit the cherries for this recipe. Serves 1–2.

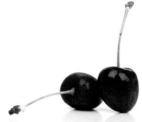

30 cherries, pitted
3 red apples
1 cup fresh blueberries
1 cup strawberries, tops removed

Juice all ingredients and serve.

FYI: Cherries

Cherries are an excellent source of calcium, phosphorus, and vitamin C. Blueberries also provide vitamin C and are an excellent laxative. They improve circulation, benefit eyesight, and have antioxidant and antibacterial properties.

ENERGIZING TONIC

This spicy drink stimulates circulation and helps rev up metabolism by creating heat and energy. I usually double or triple this recipe and keep it on hand. Pour some into ice-cube trays and freeze, then use the frozen cubes in water or tea. If you're familiar with Yogi tea or chai, this is like a minty version of those popular Indian teas.
Serves 2.

3 cups purified water
4 slices or "coins" fresh ginger root, each ¼ inch thick
4 cinnamon sticks, cut in half
1 Tbsp. dried peppermint, either loose or in a tea bag
½ tsp. cardamom seeds
⅛ tsp. whole cloves

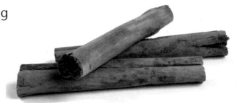

In a medium saucepan, combine all of the ingredients and simmer for about 10 minutes. Strain and drink hot or cold.

FYI: Peppermint

Peppermint reduces gas, nausea, and the spastic symptoms of irritable bowel syndrome. Caution: peppermint leaf is strictly off-limits for those who are pregnant, have gallstones, or have a hiatal hernia.

REJUVENATION TONIC

Enjoy this simple-to-make tonic in the morning, as an afternoon pick-me-up, or throughout the day as a 24-hour rejuvenating cleanse. Your cells will sizzle with enthusiasm and vitality.

Serves 2.

2 cups purified cold water
1 Tbsp. protein powder
1 Tbsp. fresh lemon juice
1–2 tsp. 100% pure organic maple syrup or raw agave nectar
⅛ tsp. organic cayenne pepper

Blend all ingredients on slow speed and serve.

Variation: You can substitute 1 cup fresh pineapple juice, coconut water, or apple juice for 1 cup of the water. Reduce sweetener if using juice.

FYI: One-Day Cleanse

One day each month (or more often), when you don't have to work and can take it easy, drink this Rejuvenation Tonic three times during the day combined with juices made from a blend of two to three vegetables and fruits (as opposed to all fruit). This is a great way to cleanse, detoxify, and rejuvenate the body, mind, and spirit. On your cleanse days, create opportunities to get extra sleep, breathe deeply, take a long bubble bath, spend time in nature, and meditate.

ANTIOXIDANT EXPRESS

This free-radical-scavenger cocktail will do wonders for boosting immunity and restoring youthful vitality.

Serves 2–3.

1 cup organic green tea, freshly brewed and chilled
4 medium carrots, washed but not peeled
1 red or green apple
½ cup broccoli sprouts
1 stalk broccoli, including florets
½ cup cauliflower
3 leaves romaine lettuce
¼ red bell pepper
¼ yellow or orange bell pepper
¼ wedge lemon (with peel, if organic) and an extra one for garnish
¼-inch piece fresh ginger root
1 Tbsp. of your favorite protein powder

Juice everything but the protein powder. After juicing is completed, blend in the powder. Serve with lemon wedge.

FYI: Green Tea

While all of the vegetables in the Antioxidant Express are rich in antioxidants, green tea takes the prize. The levels found in green tea are among the highest in any food or beverage. These body-friendly companions aid in the prevention of disease by battling free radicals, which are believed to be a major cause of cancer, heart disease, and aging. All black, white, and green teas come from the same bush. The differences exist in the different times of harvesting and different methods of processing.

NATURAL-BEAUTY COCKTAIL

Drink this daily for a week. Your skin will glow, your eyes will sparkle, and your energy will soar.

Serves 2.

1 medium red or green apple
1 sweet bell pepper (red, yellow, or orange)
3 medium carrots
3 leaves romaine lettuce
2 stalks celery
½ medium cucumber
¼ wedge lemon (with peel, if organic)
¼-inch piece fresh ginger root

Juice all ingredients and serve.

EASY SLEEPYTIME COCKTAIL

Taken an hour before bedtime, this delicious combination is guaranteed to help you fall asleep without having to count sheep.

Serves 1–2.

1 cup freshly brewed chamomile tea
2 apples
2 stalks celery
¼ cup parsley

Juice the apples, celery, and parsley, then mix with the tea. Sip slowly.

FYI: Chamomile Tea

Tea made from this mildly sedating herb is useful in treating insomnia and soothing gastritis, an inflammation of the stomach lining. Caution: Chamomile belongs to the same plant family as daisies and dandelions. If you're allergic to those plants, you should avoid chamomile.

PEACEFUL COCKTAIL

If you're feeling irritable or anxious, this colorful drink will lift your spirits and lower your stress level.

Serves 2.

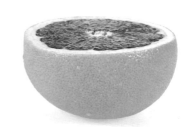

1 ruby red grapefruit, peeled (leaving pithy part on is okay)
1 pear
8 large strawberries, green tops included
¼-inch piece fresh ginger root (optional)
1 cup freshly brewed lemon-balm tea

Juice all of the fruits (and ginger, if using) and mix with the tea. As you drink this cocktail, make sure to breathe slowly and deeply.

FYI: Lemon Balm

This herb is a member of the mint family. Lemon balm is reported to help combat mild forms of anxiety and irritability. The tea also can be dabbed onto herpes sores on the mouth or genitals. Apply it three to six times a day at the first sign of an outbreak to reduce or even prevent symptoms. Some people use it as an adjunct to antiviral medications. Caution: pregnant women and people with hypothyroidism should not use lemon balm.

ANTICANCER V-12

After tasting this delicious vegetable juice, you'll never want to drink the canned varieties again.

Serves 2–3.

4 large ripe tomatoes
3 large carrots
3 stalks celery
1 sweet bell pepper (red, yellow, or orange)
4 green onions
4 leaves of the greenest romaine lettuce

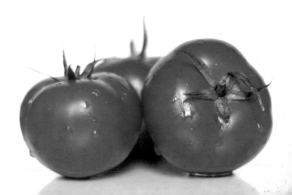

23

4 large spinach leaves
2 kale leaves
½ cup broccoli sprouts
½ small beet
⅓ cup parsley
1–3 cloves garlic (optional)
1 small lemon (with peel, if organic)
¼ tsp. sea salt

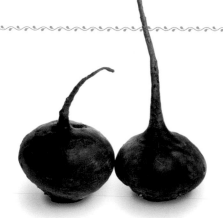

Juice all ingredients and stir in the salt. Add extra tomatoes if you need more juice.

FYI: Lutein

Lutein is a carotenoid pigment found in plants that protects the colon cells from damage caused by highly reactive compounds called free radicals. These are a type of oxygen molecule that freely moves inside cells; reacting with proteins, fats, and DNA; changing their structure and disrupting their function. Free radicals are generated by the metabolism of oxygen and other chemicals such as cigarette smoke; unsaturated fats; food additives; and environmental chemicals such as herbicides, pesticides, and preservatives. In several recent studies, eating a lutein-rich diet was reported to reduce the risk of colon cancer by as much as 17 percent. Good sources of this carotenoid include tomatoes, carrots, oranges, broccoli, kale, romaine lettuce, and spinach.

VITALITY SHAKE

I make this smoothie several mornings a week right after my workout. It really hits the spot and provides a balance of protein, carbohydrates, and omega-3 fatty acids. This smoothie is also a great meal replacement.
Serves 1–2.

1 cup purified water
1 ripe banana, peeled (I like to use a frozen banana)
½ cup frozen fruit such as blueberries, strawberries,
    cherries, peaches, raspberries, or papaya
1–2 Tbsp. protein powder
3–4 leaves romaine lettuce
1 Tbsp. flaxseed oil

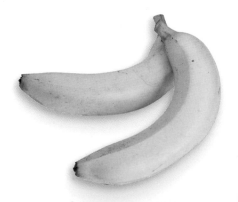

Blend, adding extra water if necessary to achieve the consistency you desire. Serve immediately.

Variation 1: Vary the fruits, and instead of water, use apple or pineapple juice, or hemp or nut milk (see Easy Nut Milk recipe that follows). To increase protein, B vitamins, and vitamin E, I add freshly milled raw wheat germ and nutritional yeast. When I want to add an extra boost of protein, I'll also blend in 6 almonds or a few pumpkin or sunflower seeds.

Variation 2: For a Vitality Dessert, pour this or another favorite smoothie into ice-cube trays and freeze. Press the frozen cubes through a Champion Juicer, and you have a very healthful sorbet-type dessert or meal.

Tip: Freezing Bananas

At any given time, I have about 20 frozen ripe bananas on hand. I use them in smoothies, to create banana ice cream (refer to the Frozen Fruit Treats recipe in Chapter 17), or simply to eat as a snack. Adding a frozen banana makes a smoothie colder and thicker. To freeze, simply peel the bananas and store whole or cut into pieces in zip-top freezer bags in your freezer.

EASY NUT MILK

This is a perfect replacement for dairy milk.
Serves 2–4.

½ cup almonds or cashews
2½ cups purified water (for soaking the nuts)

Soak the nuts in the water overnight to release and increase the nutrients and make the proteins more digestible. Drain, reserving the water. In a nut or coffee grinder or The Total Blender, grind the nuts into meal. Place the reserved water and meal in a blender and blend at high speed for about 2 minutes. Strain the resulting liquid through a fine-mesh strainer. Chill and serve.

Variation 1: Sweeten with a touch of maple, barley-malt, or brown-rice syrup or agave nectar, or add a teaspoon of pure vanilla extract.

Variation 2: For a warm drink on a chilly evening, add a dash of cinnamon, cardamom, and/or nutmeg. For a chocolate flavor, add a teaspoon of carob powder or organic raw cocoa powder. Warm on very low heat.

NUT-MILK SMOOTHIE

I always keep a quart of this in my refrigerator to enjoy with clients, family, and friends.

Serves 1.

1 cup almond-nut milk (See Easy Nut Milk recipe on previous page.)
1 ripe frozen banana, cut into chunks
Dash of cinnamon

Blend all ingredients and serve.

Variations: For a chocolate flavor, add 1 teaspoon carob powder or organic cocoa powder (I use raw powder). For a more complete, nutritious meal, blend in 1–2 tablespoons of your favorite protein powder. For a sweeter taste, blend in 3 medjool dates and a few drops of pure vanilla extract; and for an exotic taste, guaranteed to impress anyone, blend in 2 apricots with a dash of nutmeg and cardamom.

DRIED PLUM & APPLE SMOOTHIE

The more common name for dried plum is *prune,* but I don't call them that because there are so many popular misconceptions associated with the word. This is a refreshing afternoon pick-me-up guaranteed to keep you in the flow.
Serves 1–2.

1 cup vanilla nondairy yogurt
8 dried plums, pitted
½ cup frozen apple-juice concentrate (you can also
     find it bottled and unfrozen)
¼ lemon, peeled (leave pithy part on)
⅛ tsp. ground cinnamon
3 leaves fresh mint
5–6 ice cubes

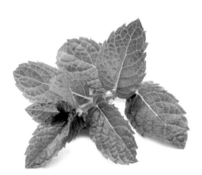

Blend until smooth and serve.

FYI: Dried Plums (Prunes)

A natural laxative, dried plums are a good source of calcium, phosphorus, potassium, beta-carotene, and iron. They help lower cholesterol and are beneficial for the blood, brain, and nerves.

CRANBERRY-APPLE COOLER

I love the unique, refreshing taste of this drink.
Serves 1–2.

12 oz. cranberry-apple juice, freshly juiced or from health-food store
1–2 Tbsp. protein powder or cashews (optional)
1 large ripe banana
Water and ice to taste (optional)

Blend all ingredients in a blender or food processor until smooth and serve.

Variations: Instead of cranberry-apple juice, try papaya, pomegranate, apple, or orange juice.

FYI: Cranberries

Cranberries have abundant antioxidant and antibacterial properties, which is why they're recommended for urinary-tract infections. They're also a good source of calcium, magnesium, potassium, manganese, and phosphorus.

CREAMY CINNAMON-BANANA SMOOTHIE

Everyone loves this smoothie!
Serves 1–2.

8 oz. vanilla almond milk (See Easy Nut Milk recipe earlier in this chapter.)
1–2 Tbsp. cashews or favorite protein powder
1 frozen or fresh ripe banana, peeled
¼ tsp. cinnamon
Pinch of nutmeg
Pinch of clove

Blend all ingredients in a blender or food processor until creamy and smooth. Serve.

FYI: Cinnamon

Researchers at Kansas State University have added cinnamon to the growing list of natural bacteria fighters. So spicing up your next glass of juice, cider, or smoothie with cinnamon may be a good idea for reasons beyond great taste.

TROPICAL-FRUIT SMOOTHIE

When you drink this smoothie, you'll feel like you're on a vacation in Hawaii. Serves 2–3.

2 ripe bananas, peeled
1 mango, peeled, seeded, and cubed
1 papaya, peeled, seeded, and cubed
1 cup fresh pineapple chunks
Ice cubes to taste

Blend all ingredients in a blender or food processor until smooth. Add water to thin out, if needed. Serve.

FYI: Bananas

Bananas provide potassium, tryptophan, vitamin C, vitamin K, and vitamin B_6. Not only do they promote sleep and remove toxic metals from the body, they also act as a mild laxative, are antifungal, and are a natural antibiotic. The pectin in bananas helps heal ulcers and lowers cholesterol. The best way to eat them is ripe—that is, when there are spots on the skin.

MIXED-MELON AMBROSIA

Melons provide a treasure trove of vitamins A, B, and C, along with trace minerals and enzymes. On a hot summer day, everyone will love this beautiful, delectable smoothie.
Serves 2–3.

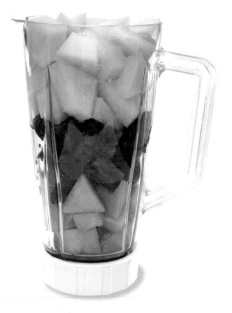

2 cups watermelon chunks
2 cups honeydew chunks
½ cup cantaloupe chunks, frozen
½ cup strawberries, frozen
1 Tbsp. maple syrup or agave nectar (optional)

Juice the watermelon and honeydew together. Pour the melon liquid into a blender and blend with the frozen fruit. Sweeten to taste.

Variation: Substitute frozen pitted cherries or blueberries for the strawberries.

FYI: Melons

Because of their high water content, melons are excellent rehydrators and cleansers. For maximum benefit, eat melons alone (don't combine with other fruits) when you're not creating a smoothie. Cantaloupe is one of the best sources of beta-carotene, potassium, and vitamin C.

MANGO-COCONUT-CREAM SMOOTHIE

Serve this smoothie in a clear glass to display its dazzling color.
Serves 2–3.

2 medium mangos (about 1 cup), peeled, seeded, and cut into chunks
1 cup orange, lemon, vanilla, or peach nondairy yogurt
¾ cup lite coconut milk (or combination of fresh coconut water and meat from a young coconut)
¾ cup vanilla hemp milk or nut milk
2 Tbsp. frozen orange-juice concentrate, thawed
Juice of ½ lime

Blend all ingredients in a blender or food processor until creamy smooth and serve immediately.

Variation: To increase protein to almost 20 grams per serving, increase nut milk to 2 cups and add 2 tablespoons of your favorite protein powder.

FYI: Coconut

Coconut contains iron, fiber, and lauric acid, an antimicrobial and antibacterial fatty acid also found in human milk. An 8-ounce serving of fresh coconut milk has only 60 calories, mostly from sugars. Try it instead of water or vegetable stock to cook grains and cereals. I drink fresh coconut water from young coconuts a few times each week.

KIWI-MELON SMOOTHIE

This combination of kiwi and melon creates a delectable taste.
Serves 2–3.

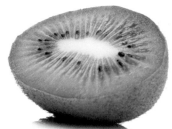

3 kiwis, peeled and cut into chunks
1 cup crenshaw, honeydew, or cantaloupe cubes, frozen
1 cup lemon, kiwi-lemon, or similar nondairy yogurt
1 cup nut milk or hemp milk
1 Tbsp. frozen orange-juice concentrate, thawed

Blend all ingredients in a blender or food processor and serve immediately.

Variations: In many smoothies that have a juice or milk base, you always have the option of using water instead. That's what I usually do unless I want the extra calories or nutrients in the liquid base. When I want more protein, I use hemp or nut milk and add 2 scoops of protein powder.

VERY STRAWBERRY-BANANA SMOOTHIE

The combination of strawberries high in vitamin C and banana that's high in potassium is a nutritional winner, and the beautiful rose color of this smoothie nourishes the soul.
Serves 2–3.

8 frozen strawberries
1 ripe frozen banana, cut into chunks
⅔ cup fresh strawberry juice
½ cup vanilla nondairy yogurt
2 Tbsp. frozen apple-juice concentrate, thawe
    (or bottled, unfrozen concentrate)
1 Tbsp. Barlean's Omega Swirl (flavored flaxseed oil)

Blend all ingredients in a blender or food processor and serve. If desired, add 1–2 scoops of protein powder to increase protein.

PEACH SMOOTHIE

What could be finer than the taste of fresh summer peaches?
Serves 3–4.

4 ripe peaches, peeled, pitted, and cut into chunks
1 ripe frozen banana, peeled and cut into chunks
1 cup vanilla or peach nondairy yogurt
1⅓ cups almond-nut milk or vanilla hemp milk
2 large ice cubes
½ tsp. pure vanilla extract

Blend all ingredients in a blender or food processor and serve immediately.
Variation: Substitute nectarines, apricots, or pears for the peaches.

FYI: Peaches

A favorite summertime treat, peaches are a good source of calcium, magnesium, phosphorus, vitamin C, potassium, beta-carotene, and folic acid. They're a mild diuretic and laxative, are very alkalizing, and are cleansing for the kidneys and bladder.

POSITIVELY PEAR SMOOTHIE

Heavenly! For best results, be sure to use ripe pears.
Serves 1–2.

1 cup pears, peeled, cut into chunks, and frozen
1 ripe frozen banana, cut into chunks
¾ cup vanilla nut milk or hemp milk

Blend all ingredients in a blender or food processor until smooth. Serve immediately.

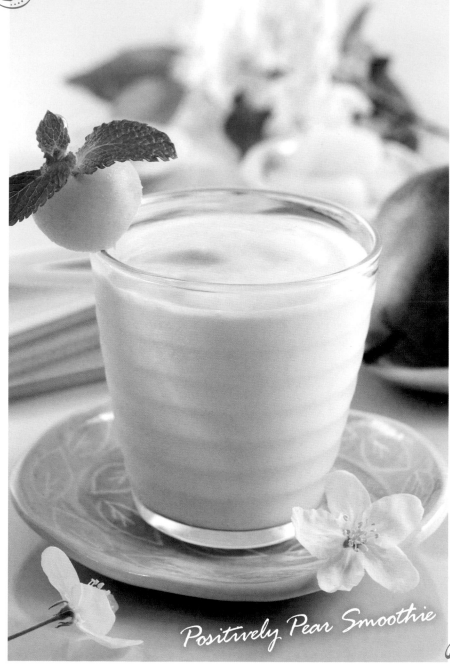

Positively Pear Smoothie

FYI: Pears

Pears are not only delicious but are also a great source of pectin, which aids peristalsis and the removal of toxins. They're a natural diuretic and are a good source of calcium, magnesium, phosphorus, potassium, beta-carotene, folic acid, and iodine, which makes them an excellent food for weight loss.

CANTALOUPE-BERRY SMOOTHIE

This satisfying, low-calorie drink contains a treasure trove of nutrients. Serves 2–3.

½ ripe cantaloupe, cut into chunks
1 cup berry nondairy yogurt
1 cup frozen berries (blueberries, strawberries, blackberries, or raspberries)
1 cup vanilla nut milk or hemp milk

Blend all ingredients in a blender or food processor and serve immediately. *Variation:* To increase protein, add 1–2 scoops of your favorite protein powder.

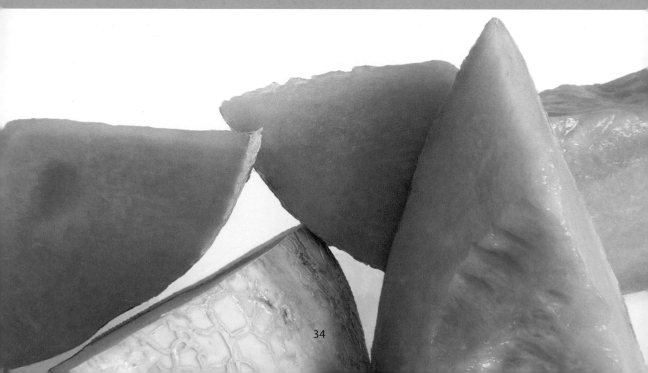

VEGGIE SMOOTHIE

Here's a great way to "eat" your vegetables! The combination of miso and mint may sound odd, but it adds a wonderful balance of flavors to this veggie drink.

Serves 3–4.

2 cups carrot juice (about 8–10 carrots)
1 cucumber, peeled if not organic
1 sweet bell pepper (red, yellow, or orange)
6 leaves romaine lettuce
3 leaves cabbage (green or purple)
⅓ cup nondairy yogurt
½ small lemon (with peel, if organic)
1–3 cloves garlic (optional)
2 Tbsp. protein powder
1 Tbsp. flaxseed oil
1–2 tsp. organic miso (sweet)
Fresh mint sprigs, for garnish

Juice enough carrots to make 2 cups of liquid. Continue to juice the other vegetables and the lemon. Pour this mixture into a blender or food processor and add the nondairy yogurt, protein powder, flaxseed oil, and organic miso. Blend all ingredients until creamy smooth. Pour into chilled glasses and garnish with a sprig of mint.

Variation: Add additional yogurt, protein powder, and miso to this juice (or any other vegetable juice you make) to create a delicious and nutritious protein salad in a glass.

FYI: Fruits, Vegetables, and Blood Pressure

Eating more fruits and vegetables helps lower high blood pressure and reduce the bone loss that leads to osteoporosis. In a recent study of more than 3,500 elderly women, it was found that those with the highest systolic pressure (the upper number in the blood pressure reading) lost almost twice as much bone mass each year as did those with the lowest systolic pressure. In other words, high blood pressure hastens bone loss, promoting calcium excretion.

CREAMY CHERRY SMOOTHIE

This beautiful smoothie really hits the spot. It will fill you up and leave you energized for hours.
Serves 2–3.

1 cup frozen pitted cherries
4–5 large ice cubes
1½ cups vanilla almond nut milk
⅓ cup lemon or vanilla nondairy yogurt
1 Tbsp. Barlean's Omega Swirl (flavored flaxseed oil)
½ tsp. pure vanilla extract
⅛ tsp. pure organic peppermint, orange, or lemon extract

Blend all ingredients in a blender or food processor until smooth and serve immediately.

WATERMELON-GINGER REFRESHER

This is one of my favorite drinks—simple, nutritious, and elegant.
Serves 3–4.

5 cups watermelon, seeded and cut into chunks
1½ Tbsp. fresh ginger root juice (put through your juicer)
1⅓ cups purified water
1 tsp. fresh lime juice
Fresh mint sprigs

Blend all ingredients in a blender or food processor and serve.
Variation: To create a "slushy" version, freeze 3 cups of watermelon chunks and blend with the remaining 2 cups of unfrozen watermelon. Pour into glasses that have been chilled in the freezer and garnish with fresh mint.

Tip: Toasted Watermelon Seeds

Remove the seeds from a watermelon, then rinse, season, and toast them for a delicious snack.

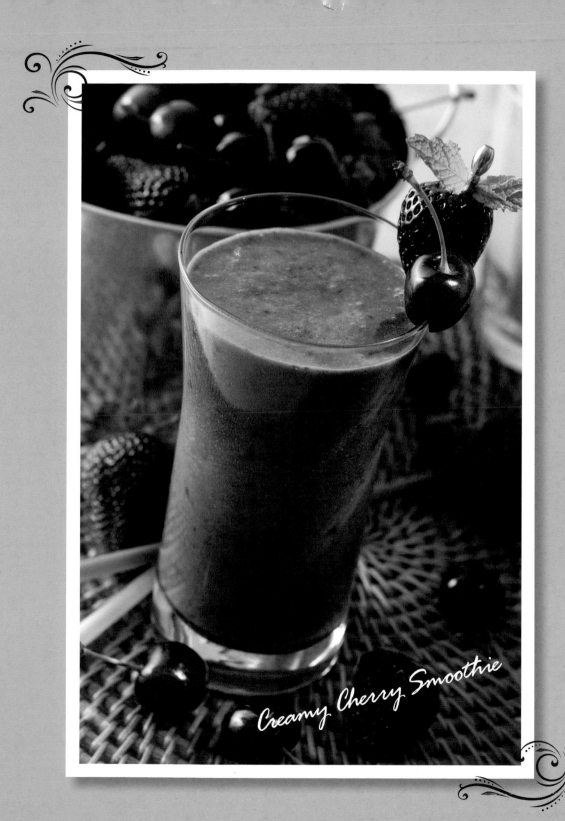

Creamy Cherry Smoothie

FRUIT POWER SHAKE

This is a great way to jump-start your day.
Serves 2–3.

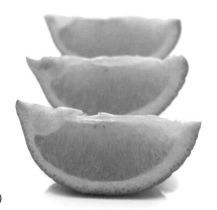

1⅓ cups fresh orange juice or apple juice
½ orange, cut into chunks (peel removed)
1 ripe banana, cut into chunks
6 frozen strawberries, green tops removed
10 frozen pitted cherries
⅓ cup apple, peeled
½ cup vanilla nut milk
1–2 Tbsp. Barlean's Omega Swirl (flavored flaxseed oil)

Blend all ingredients in a blender or food processor until smooth and serve right away.

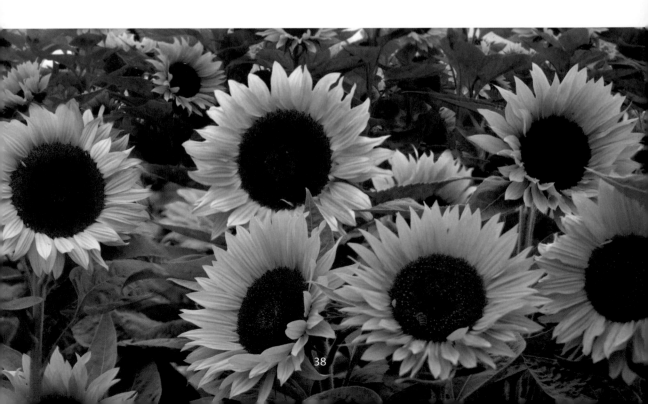

CHAPTER 3

BREAKFASTS & BRUNCHES

*"The doctor of the future will give no medicine, but
will interest his patients in the care of the human frame,
in diet, and in the cause and prevention of disease."*

— THOMAS A. EDISON

If you're like a lot of my friends, you're chronically pressed for time and feel lucky if you find a moment to wolf down a muffin and gulp some coffee on your way to the office. Unfortunately, skipping breakfast or eating empty-calorie, processed "breakfast foods" lowers metabolism and energy and sets up a body chemistry that tends to turn food into fat more easily. So if your goal is to shed some pounds, there's no more important meal than the first one of the day. A good breakfast stokes the fire and wakes your metabolic machinery out of inertia from the night's rest. When one of your goals is to accelerate fat loss, make sure you eat in the morning.

The word *breakfast* literally means "breaking a fast." If you want to start the day off right, break *your* fast with the most healthful foods possible. *Simple, light,* and *nutritious* are the keys to remember for your first meal of the day. Fresh fruit in season is one of the most nutritious options you can choose since it digests quickly, enabling you to reap its high energy benefits in a matter of minutes. Fruit is also the food with the highest water content, so it rehydrates your body and fills you up without adding lots of calories. As you adopt the habit of eating fresh fruit for your morning meal, you'll see how it helps give you an energetic start to the day without leaving you feeling stuffed.

In addition, fruit smoothies are a quick, easy, and healthful breakfast when you want to lose weight. Remember, it's best to eat several smaller meals throughout the day instead of two or three larger meals if you want to lose fat and restore youthful vitality. This is called "grazing."

In this chapter, I've included some of my favorite breakfasts. They aren't too heavy and will give you a balance of carbohydrates, protein, and essential fatty acids. (I didn't give you too many fruit dishes since they're so simple to make.) Most of the recipes that follow also will work well for weekend brunches when more food might be appropriate.

PINWHEEL CITRUS DELIGHT

This is one of my favorite breakfasts because it's as beautiful to look at as it is delicious and nutritious to eat. I always put the fruit on top of a bed of romaine lettuce in a pinwheel design and sprinkle cinnamon over all of it.

Serves 2–4.

2 ruby red grapefruit
1 large juicy navel orange
4 large ripe kiwis
8–10 hearts of romaine
Fresh berries, such as blueberries, raspberries, black raspberries,
    and strawberries
⅓ cup raw almonds, raw walnuts, and/or raw cashews (alone or combined)
Fresh mint sprigs, for garnish

Peel the fruit with a knife. Be sure to remove all of the white pith that's just under the skin of the citrus. Slice the fruit into circles, as opposed to sections. Arrange the circles of fruit on top of the romaine in a way that looks great and shows off all of the colors. Sprinkle the berries around them. In a nut grinder, coarsely grind the nuts and then mix them together in a bowl. Sprinkle 1 tablespoon of the nut mixture over each plate and garnish each one with a sprig of mint.

Variation: Try this recipe using other fruits that you love such as melons, pineapple, tangerines, papaya, mango, pears, apples, peaches, apricots, and nectarines.

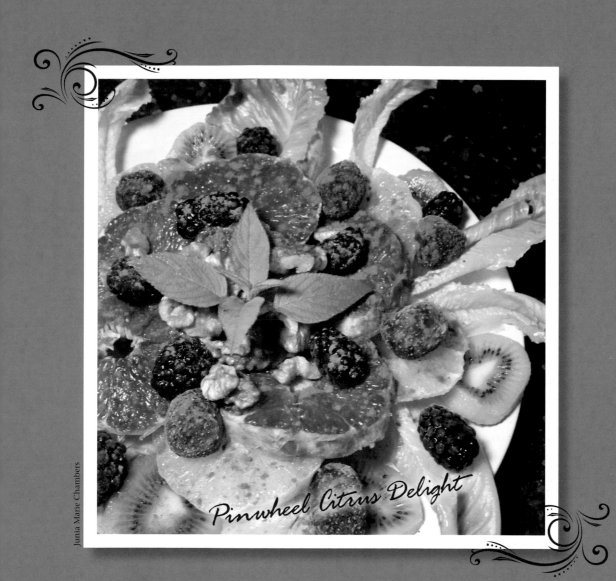

Pinwheel Citrus Delight

Junia Marie Chambers

FYI: Grapefruit

Ruby red grapefruit contains more nutrients than the white or pink varieties. A good source of vitamin C, potassium, magnesium, and calcium, grapefruit also contains salicylic acid, which helps arthritis. Grapefruit is good for allergies and infections of the throat and mouth.

BERRY SALAD WITH FRUIT SAUCE

The colors of this recipe always lift my spirits.
Serves 3–4.

3 cups fresh berries, such as blueberries, raspberries, blackberries, and
    strawberries, rinsed well
3 ripe bananas, sliced
1 Tbsp. vanilla nut milk or other nut milk
2–3 drops pure peppermint extract
Fresh mint sprigs, for garnish

In a bowl, mix 2 of the bananas with 2 cups of the berries. Blend together remaining bananas, berries, nut milk, and peppermint extract to make a sauce. Arrange fruit in the bowls (slice strawberries, if large) and top with the sauce. Be creative: drizzle the sauce in a pattern that pleases your eye and suits your own personal style. Garnish with mint sprigs.

FYI: Berries

Berries provide calcium, magnesium, phosphorus, potassium, vitamin B_3, and vitamin C. They're excellent for female reproductive health and help relieve menstrual cramps. Raspberry-leaf tea reduces nausea in pregnancy. Berries, in general, are low in calories and very nutritious, so keep your refrigerator and freezer stocked with lots of them.

MUESLI

This unroasted granola treat is very nourishing and versatile.
Serves 2–3.

5 medium apples
½ lemon
1⅓ cups rolled oats
¼ cup rye flakes
¼ cup prunes, pitted
2 medjool dates, pitted; or 3–4 regular
    soft dates, pitted
2 Tbsp. raw sunflower seeds
¼ cup walnuts or almonds
⅛ cup hemp nuts
¼ cup small raisins
Dash cinnamon

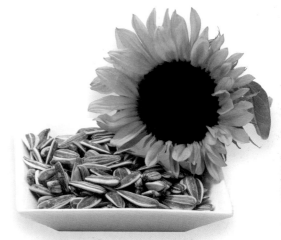

Core and quarter the apples. Juice the wedges and save 1½ cups of the juice and all of the pulp. Juice the lemon and set aside the juice. In a food processor, process oats, rye flakes, prunes, dates, seeds, nuts, raisins, and cinnamon until coarsely ground. Put this mixture in a large bowl. Add the apple pulp after discarding any large pieces of skin. Add the apple and lemon juices to the ground mixture and mix well. Let the mixture sit for about 15 minutes. Serve with fresh fruit on top, such as sliced strawberries. Also try it with vanilla nut milk or a large dollop of nondairy yogurt or applesauce.

Tip: Freezing Muesli

I often make a large batch of muesli without the apple juice or pulp and freeze it until needed. I add the liquid and apples when I'm ready to eat. Sometimes I combine the ground mixture with some nut milk or grated apple. Right before eating, I also might add some freshly milled raw wheat germ and freshly ground flaxseed.

SENSATIONAL SPICY GRANOLA

This easy-to-make recipe is perfect for those mornings when your softball team comes over for breakfast. Double the portions if the opposing team is coming, too.

Serves 12–16.

3 apples
1 small lemon
1 small orange
8 cups rolled oats
2 cups unsalted raw nuts (almonds, walnuts, pecans, cashews, pine nuts, or pistachios, or a combination)
1 cup wheat bran
1 cup wheat germ
½ cup raw, unsalted sunflower seeds
½ cup unsweetened shredded coconut
¼ cup sesame seeds
¼ cup hemp nuts
¼ cup unrefined sesame or canola oil
¼ cup brown-rice syrup
3 Tbsp. maple syrup
1 Tbsp. pure vanilla extract
1 Tbsp. apple concentrate
1 tsp. pure almond extract
2 tsp. cinnamon
1 tsp. cardamom
1 tsp. ground ginger
½ tsp. coriander
½ tsp. nutmeg
½ tsp. sea salt
1 cup chopped dried fruit (dried plums, raisins, dates, cherries, peaches, or apples, or a combination)

Preheat oven to 300° F. Juice the apples, lemon, and orange, reserving the combined juice. In a large bowl, combine the rolled oats, nuts, wheat germ and

Sensational Spicy Granola

bran, coconut, seeds, and all of the spices. In a small saucepan, stir together the combined juice, oil, maple and brown-rice syrups, apple concentrate, and vanilla and almond extracts over low heat until well blended and heated through. Pour the hot liquid over the dry mixture and combine until very well mixed. Spread the mixture on two 11" x 17" jelly-roll pans and bake for 25–30 minutes, stirring to relayer it every 5–7 minutes, or until the oats are crisp and brown but not burned. When done, remove from the oven and pour into a large, cool bowl to stop the cooking. Add the dried fruit and combine thoroughly. Set aside to cool completely. Store in an airtight container.

Tip: Storing Granola

I keep my extra granola in zip-top bags. It freezes so well that you might consider doubling or tripling the recipe so that you always have some on hand.

BANANA-APPLESAUCE MUFFINS

These make a great snack or on-the-go meal.
Makes 12 muffins.

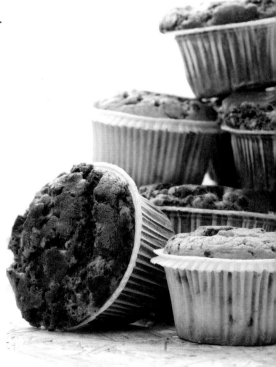

1¼ cups oat flour
1 cup rice flour
1 tsp. baking soda
½ tsp. baking powder
2 tsp. cinnamon
¼ tsp. nutmeg
1 very ripe banana
⅔ cup applesauce
½ cup apple juice
⅓ cup orange juice
1 large apple, peeled, cored, and diced
½ cup raisins

Preheat the oven to 350° F. In a large bowl, combine the flours, baking soda, baking powder, and spices. In a food processor, combine the banana, applesauce, and juice. Blend in the dry ingredients a little at a time. Transfer mixture to the large bowl and fold in the diced apple and raisins. Fill the cups of a nonstick muffin tin about ⅔ full and bake for 12–13 minutes. Serve with Apricot & Prune Spread or Apple Butter Spread (see Chapter 4).

CREAMY COCONUT MILLET CEREAL

This is a lovely change from regular oatmeal.
Serves 4.

1 cup millet
1 cup purified water
½ cup lite coconut milk
½ cup vanilla nut milk (see Chapter 2)
1 Tbsp. maple syrup
2 Tbsp. brown-rice syrup
⅓ cup unsweetened shredded coconut
⅛ tsp. cinnamon
⅓ cup raisins, chopped pitted dates, diced apples, dried cherries, or a
    combination (optional)

In a blender, process the millet until it's very fine. In a saucepan, bring water and milks (coconut and nut) to a boil. Add the millet and stir. Lower heat to a simmer and add syrups, cinnamon, and fruit. Cook until smooth and soft, about 3–5 minutes. Top with the shredded coconut and serve with vanilla nut milk. Add raisins, dates, dried apples, or dried cherries, as desired.

FYI: Millet

This gluten-free grain is highly alkaline and easily digestible. Rich in fiber and a low-allergenic food, millet is rich in magnesium, potassium, phosphorus, and vitamin B_3.

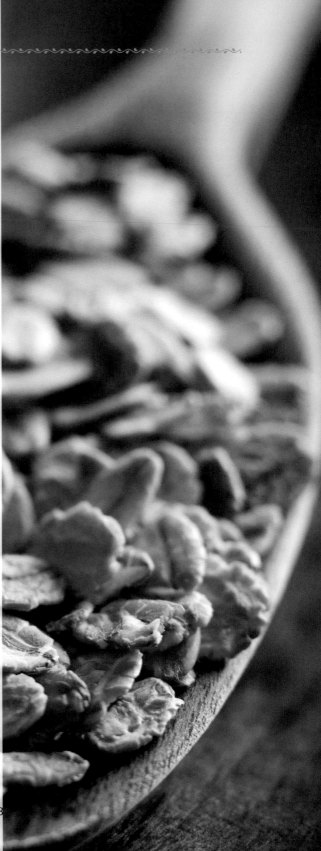

OATMEAL DELUXE

Here's one of the tastiest oatmeal recipes you'll ever make.
Serves 5–8.

5 cups purified water
¾ tsp. cinnamon
⅛ tsp. nutmeg
1 tsp. coriander
3¼ cups rolled oats
½ cup raw sunflower seeds
2 cups vanilla nut milk
   (see Chapter 2)
2 cups apples, peeled, cored,
   and grated
1 Tbsp. maple syrup
½ cup raisins, dried cherries,
   chopped dates, or a combination

In a large saucepan, combine the water, cinnamon, nutmeg, and coriander and bring to a boil. Add the remaining ingredients and reduce heat to low. Cook until thickened, stirring occasionally. Serve with warmed vanilla nut milk or other milk of your choice.

FYI: Oats

Oats, an outstanding antioxidant grain, are packed with a high fiber content, which ensures a mild laxative and cholesterol-lowering effect. Oats are excellent for bones and connective tissue because they're a good source of calcium, magnesium, and phosphorus, as well as manganese, iron, vitamin B_5, folic acid, and silicon.

TOP-OF-THE-MORNING QUINOA CEREAL

Pronounced "KEEN-wah," this versatile food is a newly rediscovered ancient grain that originated with the Incas. It has an impressive nutritional profile and a nutty, distinctive flavor. Some folks call it the "super grain." Its easy-to-digest protein, calcium, iron, potassium, magnesium, lysine, and vitamin B_3 make it a winner on any health enthusiast's menu.

Serves 4–5.

1⅓ cups quinoa
2 cups fresh apple juice
1 tsp. unrefined sesame oil
1 tsp. brown-rice syrup
⅛ tsp. sea salt
2 Tbsp. pecans, cashews, walnuts, or pistachios,
    roasted and finely chopped

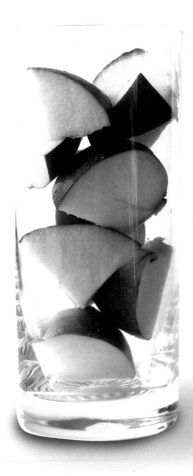

Put the quinoa in a large bowl and cover with cold water. Gently rub it between your palms for about 10 seconds to wash off the saponin, a bitter, naturally occurring substance that acts as a natural pesticide. Drain the grain in a fine-mesh strainer. Repeat this washing process 3 times, then run cold water through quinoa until the water runs almost clear.

In a medium saucepan, combine the juice, oil, syrup, and salt and bring to a boil. Make sure it doesn't boil over. Add the washed quinoa, cover, and lower the heat. Simmer for 12–15 minutes, or until all of the liquid has been absorbed. Remove from the heat and let stand for 5 minutes. Add the nuts and fluff with a fork. Serve warm or chilled. Top with vanilla nut milk, applesauce, or a dash of cinnamon.

Variations: Instead of apple juice, you can substitute orange juice, vanilla soy milk, coconut milk, rice milk, nut milk, water, or any combination.

SCRAMBLED TOFU

I love breakfast food anytime, and this great protein dish has no cholesterol. Most scrambled recipes call for sautéing. In this one, you cook everything in a light vegetable broth or water.

Serves 4.

¼ cup Vegetable Broth (see Chapter 7) or water
1 small red pepper, diced
1 zucchini (optional)
¾ cup mushrooms, diced
½ red onion, diced
½ cup green onions, finely chopped
1 clove garlic, finely minced
1 lb. firm to extra-firm silken tofu, drained, pressed dry, and crumbled
1½ tsp. curry powder (or 1 tsp. turmeric if curry is too spicy for you)
1 Tbsp. Bragg Liquid Aminos or low-sodium tamari

Set a sauté pan over high heat and add Vegetable Broth to scald. Add the vegetables, Bragg Liquid Aminos, and garlic, and sauté until tender. Add the tofu and spices, mixing everything well for about 5 minutes.

Variations: Try this recipe with different vegetables. Most vegetables work well, such as carrots, broccoli, or cauliflower. Serve with salsa and warm whole-grain pita bread to make a Tex-Mex delight. Add some roasted or hash brown potatoes, and you'll never miss eggs again.

FYI: Tofu

Made from soybeans, tofu is a vegetarian source of protein and has anticancer and cholesterol-lowering properties. Besides amino acids, it's also packed with iron, potassium, calcium, magnesium, vitamin A, and vitamin K. Some people have problems digesting soy. Personally, if I choose to eat these products, I always purchase organic versions of them or I make my own using my stellar SoyQuick Premier Milk Maker. It makes the best fresh soy milk (and rice milk) and tofu in minutes and is so easy to use and clean. Caution: If you have a history of breast cancer in your family, check with your doctor before consuming tofu and other soy products, or feeding soy formulas to your infant.

TOFU PANCAKES

This recipe is so tasty that you'll never believe it's both oil and egg free. Make these pancakes for a healthful, festive brunch.

Serves 3–4.

1 (12-oz.) package soft lite silken tofu
⅔ cup vanilla soy milk or nut milk
½ medium ripe banana
½ cup whole-wheat pastry flour
¼ cup flaxseed meal
1 Tbsp. brown-rice syrup
Dash cinnamon
Nonstick cooking spray

In a blender, combine all ingredients and blend until smooth. Heat a nonstick griddle over medium heat and lightly mist with nonstick cooking spray. Pour batter onto the hot griddle. When bubbles appear, turn the pancake over. Don't be concerned if the first couple of pancakes don't look great. They're priming the griddle for the best to come. Serve with soy yogurt, maple syrup, or applesauce.

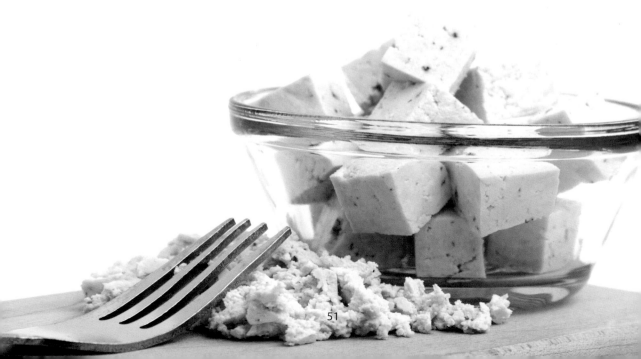

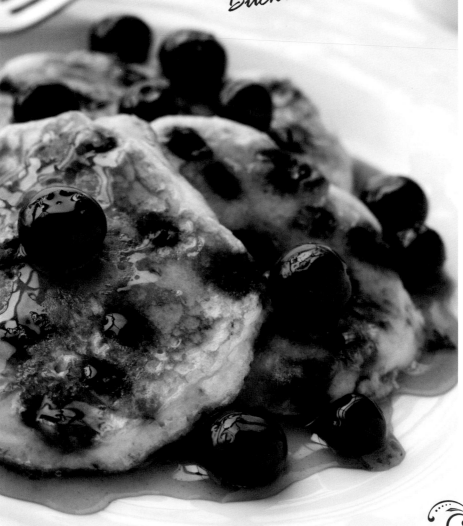

Orange-Blueberry Buckwheat Pancakes

ORANGE-BLUEBERRY BUCKWHEAT PANCAKES

The hearty buckwheat taste of these pancakes is an unexpected delight.
Serves 2–4.

¾ cup vanilla nut milk (or rice milk or soy milk)
1 Tbsp. fresh orange juice
1 tsp. orange zest (from an organic orange only)
2 Tbsp. maple syrup
1 cup buckwheat flour
⅛ tsp. sea salt
1 tsp. baking powder
Dash cinnamon
½ cup blueberries
Maple syrup, applesauce, or all-fruit preserves, for topping
Nonstick cooking spray

In a small bowl, mix together milk, syrup, orange juice, and zest. In a large bowl, mix together flour, baking powder, salt, and cinnamon. Pour liquid mixture into the dry mixture and combine, then fold in the blueberries. Lightly coat a nonstick skillet or griddle with nonstick cooking spray and set over high heat. Pour batter and cook 1–2 minutes over medium heat or until the tops of the pancakes bubble. Turn them and cook briefly on the second side. Serve with a topping of your choice.

FYI: Buckwheat

Buckwheat contains all eight essential amino acids, making it an excellent plant-based protein. It's rich in phosphorus, beta-carotene, vitamin C, calcium, magnesium, phosphorus, potassium, zinc, manganese, and folic acid. Caution: If you have skin allergies or cancer, check with your doctor before eating buckwheat.

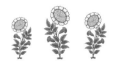

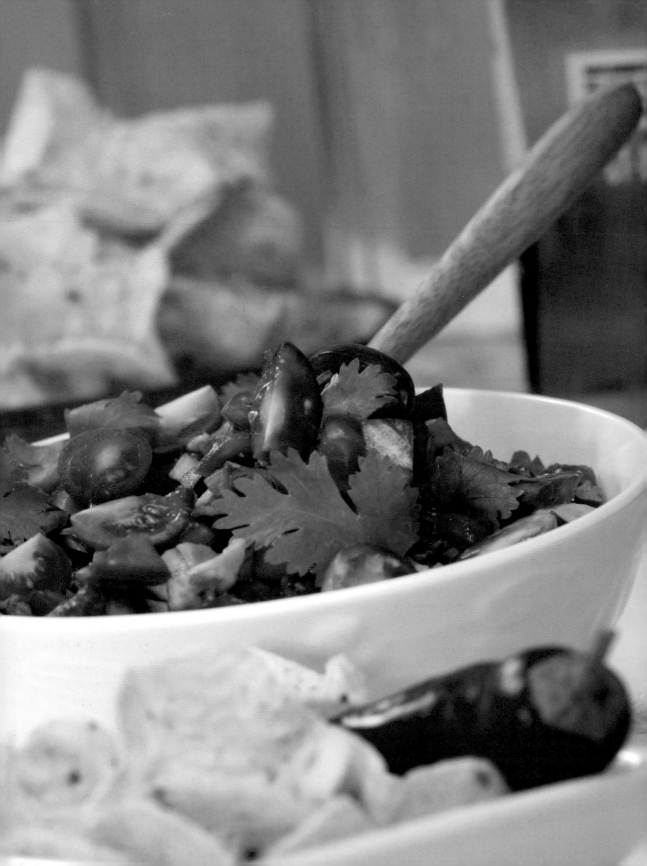

CHAPTER 4

SPREADS, SAUCES, DIPS & MARINADES

*"Have a friend over for tea. Serve cinnamon toast and
a real talk. Give the most precious gift. Give of yourself."*

— ALEXANDRA STODDARD

W hen you emphasize plant-based foods (especially leafy green vegetables) in your diet, it's helpful to have a variety of different sauces,
dips, spreads, and marinades that you can use to create a wide
range of flavors, textures, and colors. The recipes in this chapter
are easy, healthful, and delicious; and they'll allow you to create an array of
nutritious new dishes that will expand your menu repertoire. Use them often on
raw fruits and vegetables and on the Herbed Garbanzo Flatbread and the chips
in Chapter 16.

Don't be afraid to experiment by adding or subtracting a little bit of this
or that to come up with your own mouthwatering creation. Similar to making
smoothies and fresh juices, it's hard to mess up these recipes. And also as with
smoothies, you can make extra servings of your favorites. Just make sure to eat
them within three to five days. *Note:* I didn't list serving sizes on the recipes in
this section because the amounts people consume vary so much.

When you're pressed for time, you can sometimes find nonfat or low-fat
natural, bottled salad dressings—in flavors such as sweet onion, creamy garlic,
toasted sesame, zesty Italian, and Dijon—in your natural-food store. (Read the

labels carefully.) I sometimes use these dressings as dips for artichokes, baked potatoes, grains, and steamed vegetables, and in a variety of oven-roasted-vegetable recipes. If a dressing seems too watery, I stir in a small amount of ground flaxseed meal, which thickens it up nicely.

Have fun with the recipes in this chapter. They can add a lot of pizzazz to your meals. And remember that you can experiment all you want and learn to make your own healthful and delicious combinations.

APRICOT- & PRUNE-BUTTER SPREADS

These butters are great on whole-grain bread or toast, pancakes, or waffles, or as a topping for fruit. Use these spreads as a replacement for butter and oil in baking recipes.

1½ cups dried apricots and/or prunes (unsulfured)
3 cups purified water

Soak the dried fruit overnight in the purified water. In the morning, transfer the water and fruit mixture to a saucepan, adding enough additional water to cover the fruit. Simmer for 10 minutes. Strain and save the cooking water. In a food processor or blender, purée the fruit, and if necessary, blend in some of the cooking water to smooth out the texture.

Variations: To add sweetness, blend in a couple of chopped medjool dates. For some extra zing, add a dash of cinnamon or nutmeg when puréeing, add a cinnamon stick to the simmering process, or stir in lemon or orange zest at the end.

FYI: Apricots & Prunes

Apricots are rich in copper, calcium, magnesium, potassium, folic acid, vitamin C, beta-carotene, boron, and iron. They're a good laxative, potent antioxidant, and natural sweetener. Prunes (dried plums) are also a laxative and help supply calcium, phosphorus, potassium, beta-carotene, and iron.

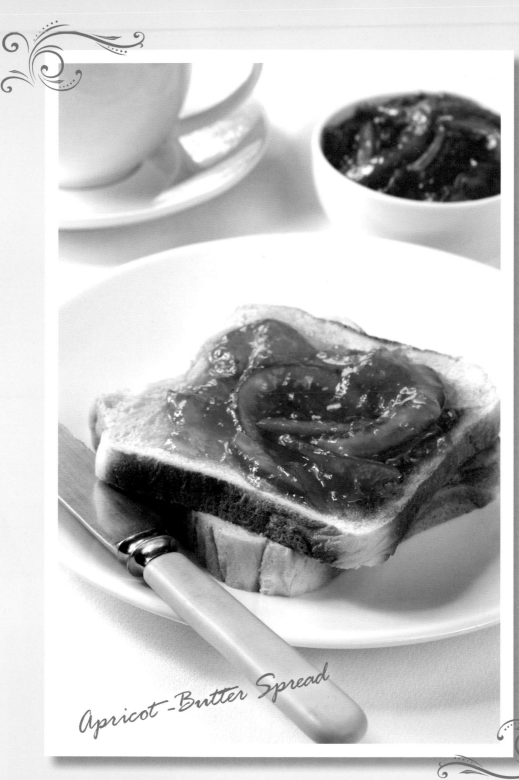

Apricot-Butter Spread

APPLE-BUTTER SPREAD

Try this healthful topping on whole-grain toast, pancakes, waffles, muffins, or fruit. You can also use this delicious spread in place of oil and eggs in your baked goods to lower fat.

6 medium apples (organic, if possible)
Purified water
Dash sea salt

Peel, quarter, and core the apples. Grate them into a heavy stockpot and add a pinch of sea salt and enough water to barely cover the grated apples. Simmer over low heat for 2 hours, or until the mixture is thick and deep brown in color, stirring occasionally to prevent burning.

Variation: Try adding some ground cinnamon, cloves, nutmeg, or allspice.

FYI: Apples

Eating an apple a day will most definitely help keep the cardiologist away. Current studies suggest that eating apples regularly reduces risk of stroke and the chances of dying from a heart attack. Apples help lower total cholesterol and triglycerides. They also provide quercetin, which may inhibit prostate, lung, and liver cancer. And because of their high antioxidant activity, apples improve brain function and memory, too. My favorite apple is the Fuji, but I also enjoy Gala, Golden Delicious, Granny Smith, Jonagold, Pink Lady, Braeburn, and Red Delicious. (Red Delicious are the highest in antioxidants.)

Tip: Apples

Apples can help ripen stone fruit, as well as other unripe fruit such as kiwis. Simply place the fruit you wish to ripen in a loosely closed paper bag at room temperature, along with an apple. The apple will release ethylene gas, which accelerates ripening.

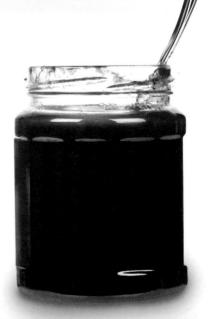

DATE-APPLE-BERRY-BUTTER SPREAD

This sweet fruit butter spread can be made more quickly than the preceding one and is especially favored by those who prefer to eat more raw, living foods, as I do. I triple the recipe so that I have lots on hand to use as a topping, spread, or simple snack.

2 apples
⅓ cup blueberries, strawberries, raspberries, or a combination
⅔ cup purified water (you may need a little extra)
1 cup pitted dates (I use medjool)
Dash of cinnamon

In a blender, combine all ingredients and pulse/blend to desired consistency. Chill before serving.

Variations: Adjust the amount of water in this recipe depending on how you're going to eat it. For example, if you're using it as a sauce to spoon on top of whole-grain pancakes or to drizzle over fresh fruit, you might want to add a little extra water. If you're using it as a spread on toast; crackers; or pear, apple, or banana slices, a little less water will keep it a bit thicker.

FYI: Pectin

Pectin, a phytochemical found in abundance in apples and other fruits, is a type of fiber that has been shown to be effective in lowering cholesterol levels.

CARROT-TAHINI SPREAD

This easy-to-prepare, colorful spread is delicious on sandwiches, on top of whole-grain toast, or as a dip for raw vegetables.

4 cups carrots, cut into 1-inch pieces (baby carrots work well, too)
¾ cup purified water
1¼ tsp. kuzu (available at natural-food or Asian specialty stores)
1–4 Tbsp. tahini

In a steamer, steam carrots for 10–15 minutes or until tender. Reserve the liquid. In a food processor or blender, purée the carrots until smooth, adding ½ cup of the cooking liquid. In a small bowl, mix kuzu in ¼ cup cold water. Add it to the carrot purée and reheat it until the mixture thickens and bubbles. Stir in the tahini. Set aside to cool.

Variations: Instead of carrots, substitute butternut squash; acorn squash; or combinations of carrots, parsnips, onions, garlic, and cabbage.

Tip: Tahini

The possibilities of tahini are endless. Traditionally used in hummus, the rich nutty flavor and creamy texture of tahini (which tastes terrific combined with lemon juice) make it an essential kitchen ingredient. The raw variety is far more delicious than roasted and can be found at your local natural-food store. Other nutritious nut and seed butters include: almond, cashew, sunflower, hemp, and pumpkin. They all make excellent replacements for peanut butter.

VEGGIE-MILLET SPREAD

Looking for a tasty spread to serve with tabbouleh or hummus or to stuff in celery, bell peppers, or Belgian endive? This highly alkalizing, health-promoting spread is perfect.

½ cup cooked millet
½ cup firm silken tofu
½ cup grated carrot
2 Tbsp. grated zucchini
2 tsp. flaxseed oil
2 Tbsp. fresh parsley, minced
1½ Tbsp. light yellow miso
1 Tbsp. almond or cashew butter
2½ Tbsp. nutritional yeast

In a blender or food processor, blend together the tofu, oil, yeast, nut butter, and miso. Pour into a bowl and combine with the remaining ingredients. Serve with warmed whole-grain pita triangles.

FYI: Nutritional Yeast

Nutritional, or brewer's, yeast, is a rich source of B vitamins, chromium, selenium, all of the essential amino acids, manganese, choline, inositol, potassium, and PABA. It can be added to sauces, dips, spreads, smoothies, soups, or breads, or sprinkled on grains and salads. When you desire a "cheesy" taste but don't want dairy, this ingredient works well. I sprinkle it on popcorn.

QUICK HIGH-PROTEIN BEAN-TOFU SPREAD

This versatile spread can be flavored any number of ways. Try it on raw vegetables, whole-grain crackers, or breads.

2 cups beans, cooked and mashed (black, navy, lentils, garbanzo, pinto, and/or split peas)
1 (12.3-oz.) package of firm lite silken tofu
Seasoning to taste

In a food processor, combine all ingredients and mix until smooth. Some of my favorites seasonings include Bragg Liquid Aminos, roasted garlic, chopped parsley, cayenne, dill, thyme, sea salt, tamari, shoyu, celery seed, and miso.

Variations: The possibilities are endless, so be creative. Blend in 2 tablespoons of tahini; sunflower-seed, almond, or cashew butters; sautéed garlic and onions; roasted bell peppers; or garlic. You also can blend in ground, unsalted pistachios, Living Harvest Hemp Nuts, steamed carrots, celery, parsnips, squash, or olives.

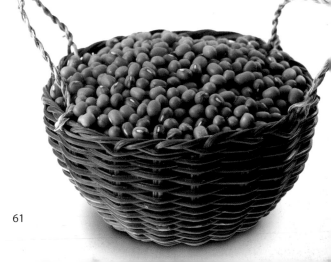

ARTICHOKE DIP

In the mood for artichoke hearts? Here's a simple, gourmet mouthwatering spread/dip that will be a guaranteed hit at any party or family gathering.

1 package frozen artichoke hearts, thawed
1 cup tofu
2 Tbsp. tahini
Dash of shoyu or low-sodium tamari

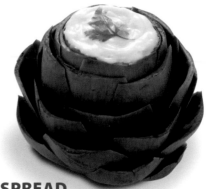

Blend all ingredients, adding water if necessary. Serve.

LEMONAISE SPREAD

This is a wonderful, light spread to use in place of mayonnaise in dips, spreads, or dressings, or on sandwiches made with whole-grain bread. Make it thick and use it as a spread, or thin and use it as a dressing, drizzled over steamed asparagus or broccoli florets.

Juice of 1 medium lemon
¼ cup cold-pressed walnut oil
¼ cup agar flakes
2 Tbsp. purified water
⅛ tsp. sea salt
Dash of cayenne and/or garlic powder (optional)

In a blender or food processor, combine all ingredients and blend to desired thickness. You can add water or oil to create the consistency you want. Refrigerate.

Variations: To make an herbed lemonaise spread, add any of your favorite herbs such as rosemary, thyme, parsley, dill, tarragon, cumin, chili powder, turmeric, curry, or herbes de Provence. To make garlic lemonaise, add pressed garlic to taste.

TOFU-CILANTRO "CREAM" SAUCE

If you want to jazz up baked potatoes, steamed vegetables, whole grains, or organic leafy greens, drizzle this sauce as you lovingly toss.

1 lb. soft tofu (organic silken works best)
¼ cup fresh cilantro, minced
¼ to ½ cup plain nut milk, soy milk, or hemp milk
2 cloves garlic, minced
1 green onion, minced
1 tsp. fresh lime juice
¼ tsp. nutritional yeast
Dash sea salt

Blend ingredients in a blender or food processor. Begin with ¼ cup milk and add a little more at a time, as needed, to get the consistency you desire.

Variations: Instead of cilantro, substitute fresh dill, basil, parsley, or even some mint.

FYI: Soybeans

A phytochemical called *genistein,* an isoflavone present in soybeans, soy flour, tofu, and textured soy protein, helps reduce blood cholesterol and fights cancer. It also may ease menopausal problems, including hot flashes, and may help in building bone density. I only eat organic tofu, soy milk, and other soy products—and only very sparingly. Note that some people have a difficult time digesting soy-based products.

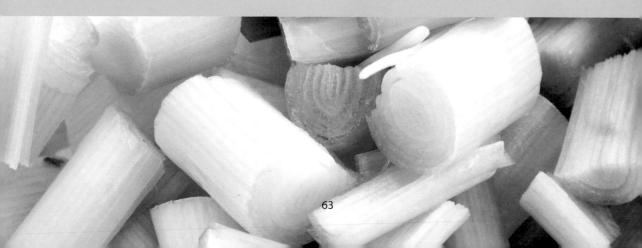

QUICK & EASY ONION DIP

This dip goes especially well with raw vegetables—cauliflower, carrots, bell peppers, and broccoli florets.

1⅓ cups plain nondairy yogurt
¼ cup sweet onion, minced
1 tsp. onion powder
1 Tbsp. green onion, minced
2 tsp. fresh parsley, minced
1 tsp. fresh lemon juice
1 tsp. lemon zest (from an organic lemon only)
2 tsp. flaxseed oil
Sea salt to taste

In a blender or food processor, combine all ingredients and blend to desired thickness. You can add water or oil to create the consistency you want. Refrigerate.

FYI: Onions

Long regarded as a super health food, onions are antiseptic, antispasmodic, anti-inflammatory, and antibiotic. They help detoxify and remove heavy metals and parasites from the body. Whether sweet or not, onions provide us with calcium, magnesium, phosphorus, potassium, beta-carotene, folic acid, and quercetin. The last nutrient, quercetin, found in red and yellow onions and broccoli, fights cancer, viruses, bacteria, and fungi. This antioxidant bioflavonoid also lowers cholesterol and reduces the risk of blood clots. If you don't digest onions very well, try small amounts and chew thoroughly. Sweet onion is usually better tolerated.

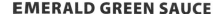

EMERALD GREEN SAUCE

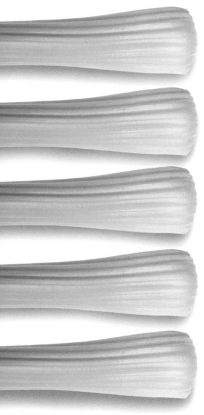

Are you looking for a healthful, colorful sauce that even kids love? Try this flavorful one on mashed potatoes, steamed vegetables, grains, or noodles, or thicken it up with blended tofu or yogurt and use it as a dip for raw or lightly steamed cold vegetables.

4 large stalks celery
¼ lb. baby leaf spinach
⅓ cup nut or hemp milk
1 Tbsp. raw, unsalted cashews
1 Tbsp. sunflower seeds
1 Tbsp. yellow or white miso
1 tsp. nutritional yeast

Juice the celery and spinach. Reserve ⅔ cup of the combined juice. If you need more, juice extra celery. In a blender or food processor, purée all ingredients, including juice, until smooth and creamy. Transfer to a saucepan and bring to a boil, stirring constantly. Lower the heat and simmer, stirring occasionally, for about 2–3 minutes. If you'd like a thinner sauce, add extra nut milk. If you'd like it thicker, blend in soft organic silken tofu, nondairy yogurt, or more cashews.

FYI: Spinach

Spinach helps regulate blood pressure, boosts the immune system, and supports bone health. It's rich in beta-carotene, folic acid, potassium, iron, vitamin B_6, vitamin C, calcium, magnesium, and the phytochemical lutein. Also found in abundance in kale and collard greens, lutein is an antioxidant carotenoid with more power than its better-known cousin beta-carotene. It fights free radical damage and has been shown to reduce the risk of macular degeneration, a common cause of blindness in older people.

HOMEMADE SUNNY KETCHUP

Unlike most store-bought ketchup, this easy-to-prepare and satisfying condiment is low in sodium and sugar, and it's fat free. You may want to double or triple the recipe. It also makes a lovely gift when you put it in a beautiful glass jar with a ribbon around the top.

12 oz. organic tomato paste
½ cup purified water
½ cup fresh organic tomato juice
2 Tbsp. fresh apple juice
1–2 cloves garlic, minced
1 tsp. nutritional yeast
2 tsp. apple-cider vinegar
½ tsp. onion powder
⅛ tsp. dried oregano

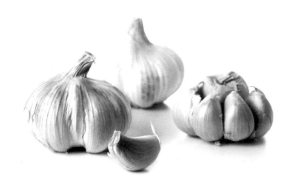

Combine all ingredients thoroughly. Store in a covered container in the refrigerator.

Variation: Add chopped fresh herbs such as cilantro, parsley, basil, or tarragon to give it a different flavor.

FYI: Tomatoes

Tomatoes are an excellent source of the phytonutrient lycopene, which has antioxidant properties, protects against cancer (notably prostate and pancreatic cancers), and stimulates the brain. All tomato products such as ketchup, tomato sauce, and tomato paste also are rich in lycopene.

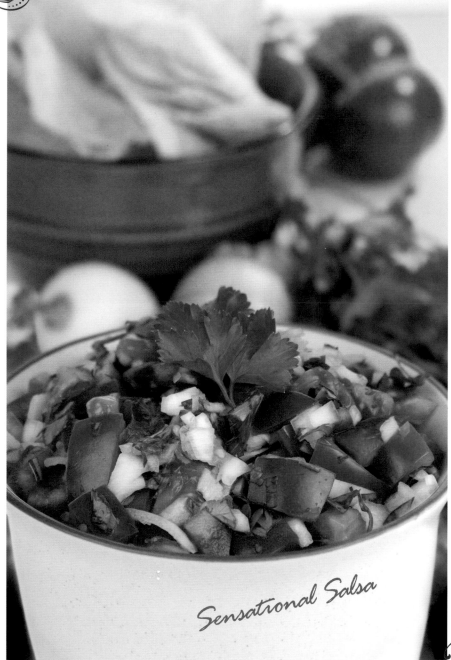

Sensational Salsa

SENSATIONAL SALSA

Besides enjoying salsa as a dip for tortilla chips and raw vegetables and in a variety of Tex-Mex dishes, I use it as a topping on everything—baked potatoes, steamed vegetables, brown rice, millet, and quinoa. I also wrap it in lettuce leaves with some avocado slices, grated carrots, and other vegetables.

1½ cup tomatoes, diced, organic if possible
2 Tbsp. finely diced white onion
1 Tbsp. finely diced red bell pepper
1 Tbsp. finely diced yellow bell pepper
1 Tbsp. fresh cilantro, chopped
2 tsp. fresh lime juice
1 jalapeno pepper, seeds and white ribs removed, minced
1 tsp. minced or pressed garlic
⅛ tsp. minced ginger
Sea salt to taste

Combine all ingredients thoroughly in a bowl. Refrigerate until ready to serve. I usually add the sea salt just before eating since it draws out the tomato juices.

Variations: For corn salsa, add ½ cup corn kernels cut right off the cob. For mango salsa, add ½ cup diced mango. For avocado salsa, add ½–¾ cup diced avocado.

Tip: What Makes Chilis Hot?

Most of the chilis' heat is in the white tissue (the ribs), and not the seeds as most people think. If you want a hotter salsa, leave in the white tissue and seeds and mince the whole thing. I recommend wearing gloves when you do this and keeping your fingers out of your eyes.

SHIITAKE MUSHROOM SAUCE

You'll find scores of ways to use this fat-free, delicious sauce, such as drizzled on whole-grain pasta or noodles, spooned over tofu steaks, or spread on top of vegetables or grain burgers.

¼ cup fresh potato juice (Yukon Gold or Finnish potato are best, but
    any kind will do.)
1 cup fresh carrot juice (4–6 carrots)
⅓ cup fresh spinach juice
2¼ cups shiitake mushrooms, cleaned and thinly sliced
1 Tbsp. low-sodium tamari
2 tsp. nutritional yeast

In a saucepan, combine the mushrooms with the three juices. Stir constantly as you bring it to a boil, then lower heat to simmer, stirring occasionally until the juice has just thickened and the mushrooms are tender. At the last moment, add the tamari and yeast and stir.

Variation: Substitute other mushrooms for the shiitakes and add your favorite herbs, such as basil, rosemary, sage, or thyme.

FYI: Mushrooms

Mushrooms help thin the blood, boost immunity, and lower cholesterol. Shiitake mushrooms contain a potent anticancer element and are rich in calcium, iron, magnesium, vitamins B_3 and B_5, folic acid, and zinc.

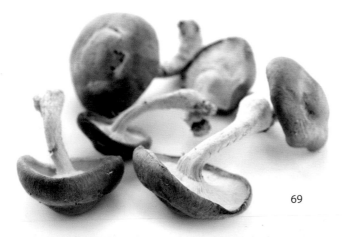

GREAT GUACAMOLE

This is one of my favorite toppings for baked potatoes, sweet potatoes, yams, salads, and grains. I also use it as a dip for raw and steamed vegetables. Leave the avocado pit in the guacamole to keep it green even when serving. Store the guacamole in the refrigerator in an opaque, airtight container with the pit in the center.

3 ripe avocados, peeled and mashed
1 small red onion, minced and lightly sautéed
3 cloves garlic, minced and lightly sautéed
¼ cup chopped green onions
⅓ cup chopped fresh cilantro
1 jalapeno pepper, finely minced
⅓ cup tomato, chopped
3 Tbsp. fresh lime juice
⅛ tsp. lemon zest
½ tsp. sea salt to taste

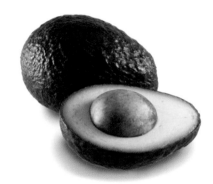

In a small bowl, mix all ingredients thoroughly and serve immediately. If you like your guacamole mild, discard the seeds and white ribs of the jalapeno pepper before mincing; if you like it hot, mince the whole thing. Be sure to wear gloves.

Variation: While you certainly don't have to sauté the onion and garlic, if you have the time, it gives the dish a wonderful flavor. I sauté using a few drops of olive oil.

FYI: Avocado

Technically a fruit, the magnificent avocado has gotten a bum rap as a fatty food that should be avoided by those desiring to lose weight. Even though 88 percent of an avocado's calories come from fat, it's primarily monounsaturated fat, which accounts for its buttery texture. It has an abundance of nutrients, including iron; copper; phosphorus; potassium; beta-carotene; folic acid; vitamins B_3, B_5, and E; and protein. Avocados are easily digested, are good for the blood, and help prevent anemia. If rapid or high weight loss is your goal, limit your avocados to only a quarter at a time (daily), eating no more than one whole avocado each week.

FESTIVE BLACK-BEAN DIP

Easy to prepare, and everyone loves it—warm or cold.

2 cups cooked black beans
1 cup grated nondairy jalapeno cheese
3 cloves garlic, pressed
3 green onions, minced
2 tsp. chopped fresh cilantro
2 tsp. ground cumin
1 tsp. Bragg Liquid Aminos, low-sodium tamari, or shoyu

In a bowl, combine all ingredients and serve warm with tortilla chips and salsa.

FYI: Black Beans

Also called the black turtle bean, black beans are an excellent source of protein and soluble fiber, which helps lower cholesterol and normalize blood-sugar levels. Add them to your salads to increase protein and turn your salad into a main course. (Don't worry about warming them up.)

SPICY & QUICK NONFAT BEAN DIP

Salsa adds a brightly flavored note and lovely color to this bean dip.

2 cups (one 16-oz. can) nonfat black beans, pinto beans, or a combination
    of both, drained and mashed
⅔ cup salsa (see recipe earlier in this chapter)

Place beans and salsa in a food processor and blend/pulse to desired consistency.

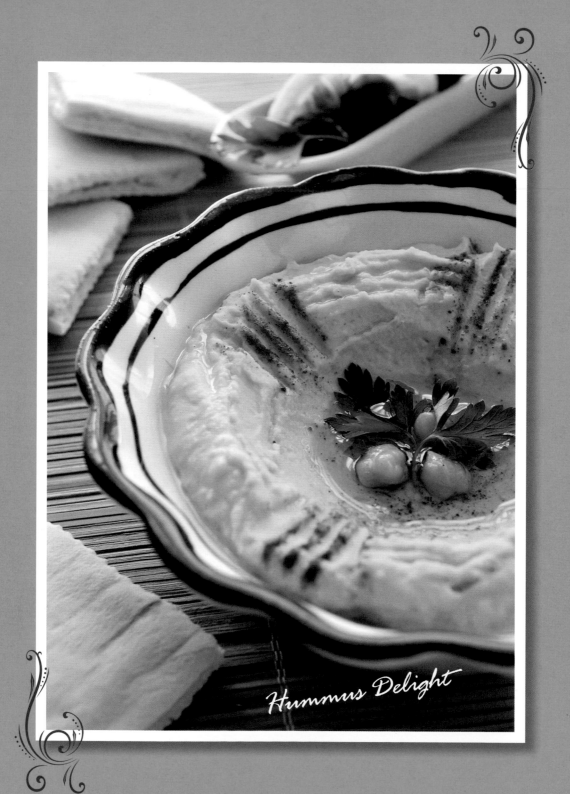

Hummus Delight

Tip: Bean Dips

It's too bad that commercial bean dips turn a low-fat, high-fiber nutritious treat into a lard-filled, artery-clogging junk food with 60 percent (or more) calories from fat. You can buy fat-free mashed beans at your natural-food store, but it's so easy to make your own. Try stuffing them in celery or Belgian endive, or using them as a dip for vegetables or baked tortillas or as a topping on grains and salads.

HUMMUS DELIGHT

Most hummus recipes call for tahini, which tastes great, but it does contain a lot of fat. I don't think you'll miss it in this recipe. I love hummus as a spread on toasted whole-grain bread with a slice of tomato, onion, and lettuce or sprouts, or wrapped in romaine lettuce leaves with grated carrots and sprouts.

2 cups garbanzo beans (chickpeas), fresh cooked or canned (reserve the liquid)
2 Tbsp. plus 1 tsp. fresh lemon juice
1–2 cloves garlic, pressed or finely minced
¼ tsp. ground cumin
1 Tbsp. minced red onion
2 Tbsp. minced fresh parsley
¼ tsp. sea salt
Cayenne pepper to taste
Fresh cracked pepper to taste

In a food processor, blend the chickpeas, lemon juice, garlic, and cumin with some of the reserved liquid. Add parsley and red onion and season with salt and pepper. Pulse briefly to mix. Keep refrigerated until ready to serve.

Variations: For black-bean hummus, add ½ cup black beans to the recipe when blending. For roasted-red-pepper hummus, add ½ cup roasted red pepper to the recipe. For roasted-garlic hummus, add 3 tablespoons roasted garlic. For roasted-onion hummus, add ⅓ cup roasted onion and 1 tablespoon of fresh chives, minced. For dill-roasted-yellow-pepper hummus, add 3 tablespoons fresh minced dill and ½ cup roasted yellow pepper. For spicy hummus, add 1 jalapeno pepper, minced, and ⅛ tsp. cayenne. To any of the above recipes, add ¼–½ cup tahini if you want a richer taste and don't mind the extra fat or calories (see Chapter 16).

FYI: Garbanzo Beans

Garbanzo beans are a very good source of calcium, magnesium, phosphorus, potassium, zinc, manganese, beta-carotene, and folic acid, as well as an excellent source of protein. They help support kidney function and cleanse the digestive system.

Tip: Cooking Beans

Beans aren't a spur-of-the-moment item. You have to remember to soak them, and it can take an hour or more for them to cook all the way through. Once a month, I prepare a large batch of garbanzo beans and store them in the freezer in freezer bags or other containers so that I never run out. I always have a ready supply whenever I want to make hummus. I also like to sprinkle whole, cooked garbanzo beans on top of my salads or mix them with my grains.

CANNELLINI-BEAN SPREAD

This is a healthful, versatile, high-protein spread that can be used for raw and steamed veggies, whole-grain crackers, and bread. It can also be rolled up in Boston or romaine lettuce leaves with grated or julienned vegetables.

1 lb. cannellini beans (about 2½ cups dry), cooked (reserve ⅓ cup liquid)
¼ cup flaxseed oil
½ cup mashed ripe avocado
⅓ cup fresh lemon juice
¼ cup tahini
2 cloves garlic, pressed
2 Tbsp. Bragg Liquid Aminos, low-sodium tamari, or shoyu
2 Tbsp. minced fresh parsley
¼ tsp. ground cumin
½ tsp. onion powder

Mash beans in a blender or food processor, then blend in remaining ingredients. Chill before serving.

Variation: For a lighter, sweeter, and higher-protein spread, add ½ cup cooked, mashed sweet potatoes and 4 oz. of organic, firm silken tofu.

QUICK & EASY FAT-FREE
ROASTED-GARLIC MARINARA SAUCE

I use this sauce in a variety of dishes and also as a salad dressing. It freezes well in zip-top freezer bags (1½ cup size works well), so you can make extra to have on hand.

½ cup Vegetable Broth, store-bought or homemade (see Chapter 7)
2 onions, chopped
3 cloves garlic, minced
2 cans (28 oz.) diced organic tomatoes or
    crushed tomatoes in purée
½ cup tomato paste
½ tsp. cayenne
½ tsp. dried oregano
½ cup roasted garlic
Sea salt and freshly ground pepper to taste

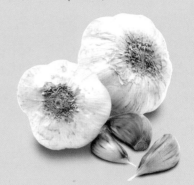

In a large skillet or stockpot, bring the Vegetable Broth to a boil over medium-high heat. Add the onion and minced garlic and sauté just until the onion is tender, about 5 minutes. Add tomatoes, tomato paste, oregano, and cayenne. Stir and bring to a boil. Reduce heat to a gentle simmer, stirring occasionally as it thickens, about 10–12 minutes. Midway through, add the diced roasted garlic. Season to taste.

Variation: I often add frozen artichoke hearts; sliced mushrooms; diced bell peppers; lightly sautéed broccoli and/or cauliflower florets; or diced squash, zucchini, and carrots to the basic recipe for a little variety.

Tip: Frozen Artichoke Hearts

Look for artichoke hearts in the freezer section of the supermarket. These are fat free and much healthier than artichoke hearts packed in oil. Keep a few packages on hand to throw in salads and to use in sauces, grains, soups, and dips.

APRICOT-GINGER CHUTNEY

Chutneys are traditionally sweet and spicy and used in India with meats and grains. I enjoy this mixture of flavors to accompany grains and salads, and even as a dip for vegetables.

1 lb. dried apricots (unsulfured), chopped into uniform pieces
4½ cups purified hot water
1½ cups apple-cider vinegar
½ cup chopped sweet onion
¼ cup garlic, chopped
3 Tbsp. chopped crystallized ginger
1 Tbsp. curry powder
¼ tsp. lemon zest (from an organic lemon only)
⅛ tsp. sea salt
1 cup organic raisins

In a large bowl, soak the apricots in hot water overnight or for at least 2 hours. After soaking, transfer fruit and liquid to a medium saucepan. Bring the water and apricots to a boil and add remaining ingredients except the raisins. Reduce heat to low and simmer until the mixture is thick, about 15–20 minutes. Add the raisins and simmer for another 15–20 minutes, stirring occasionally, making sure the chutney doesn't stick. Cool and store in refrigerator.

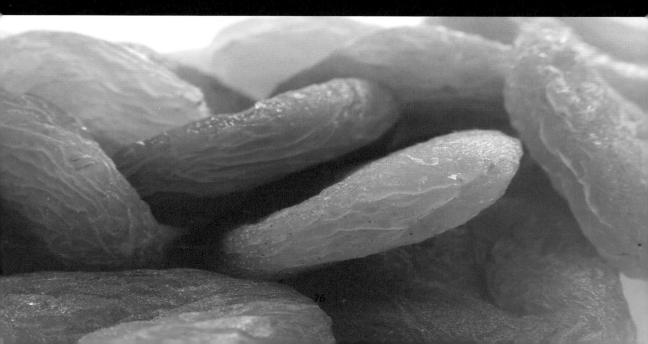

MISO-GINGER-TAHINI SAUCE

For an exotic and winning taste, spoon this sauce over Japanese udon or soba (buckwheat) noodles or drizzle over steamed vegetables, grain dishes, or potatoes.

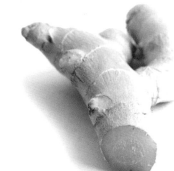

4 Tbsp. white miso
3 Tbsp. tahini
⅓ cup Vegetable Broth (see Chapter 7) or water
2 Tbsp. brown-rice vinegar
1½ Tbsp. fresh ginger juice
1 Tbsp. mirin (rice wine)
1–2 cloves garlic, pressed
½ tsp. fresh lemon juice

In a medium saucepan, combine miso and tahini. Add the rest of the ingredients and bring to a simmer, making sure it doesn't boil. Add extra water or broth if too thick or to achieve desired consistency. Serve hot or warm.

Tip: Mirin

Quality mirin is an ambrosial cooking wine, brewed and fermented from sweet rice, koji, and water. I use it in vinaigrettes, marinades, vegetable dishes, sauces, and dips.

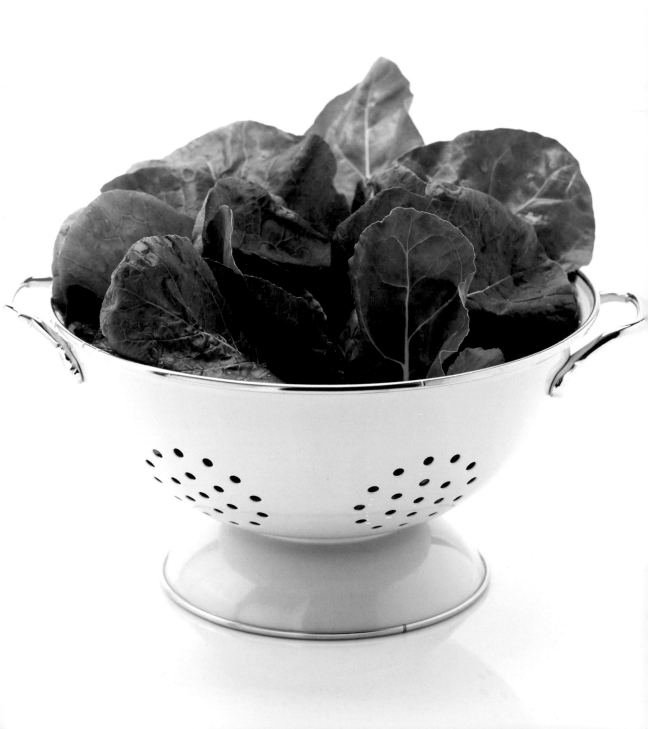

CHAPTER 5

SALADS

*"There is absolutely no substitute for greens in the diet!
If you refuse to eat these 'sunlight energy' foods, you are
depriving yourself, to a large degree, of the very essence of life."*

— H. E. KIRSCHNER, M.D.

Gone are the days when salad meant a wedge of iceberg lettuce and a few pale pink excuses for tomatoes. Hallelujah! An almost infinite variety of textures, flavors, and colors can be combined to make salads these days. And the more creative you are, the more packed with nutritional benefits your salads can be. They're easy to make, and unless you drown them in high-fat dressings, they're generally low in calories. They provide lots of fiber, enzymes, chlorophyll, vitamins, minerals (especially calcium), and antioxidants. I encourage you to eat at least one or two salads every day. They help fill you up without filling you out. Leafy greens are rich in high-quality protein per calorie compared to most foods, but since they're low in overall calories (in the quantities that most people eat), you can increase the protein content of your salads by adding beans, grains, seeds, and nuts. I like to add fresh-ground flaxseed to my salads to increase fiber and omega-3s.

Instead of having a small salad as part of your meal, get in the habit of making the salad your *entire* meal. Use a large, attractive bowl; let your imagination go; and create a masterpiece.

It's well known that most plant-based foods not only help maintain a healthy weight, but they also may aid in preventing cancer and heart disease. Here are a few of the best foods that may help prevent both diseases and are easy to bring into your salad meals several times a week: spinach; broccoli; garlic; onions; beans; carrots; flaxseed oil and freshly ground meal; beans such as garbanzo, black, kidney, and fresh soybeans (edamame); grains such as quinoa, millet, and brown rice; tomatoes; and most greens, such as romaine lettuce.

Healthful Salad Tips

Here are some tips to help make the most of your salad greens:

1. Always purchase greens as fresh as possible, without blemishes, bruises, or discoloring. They're at their best the same day you buy them, so don't store them for more than two to three days. If you have more than you know you'll eat, juice or blend them into your smoothies. Discard any pieces with signs of yellowing or discoloring. Whenever you can buy organic, do so.

2. Choose a variety of greens in different shades. Romaine lettuce packs eight times the vitamin A of iceberg lettuce. Arugula has more than twice the calcium of milk, cup for cup. A half cup of spiky dandelion leaves provides 78 percent of your daily value of vitamin A. One cup of spicy baby mustard greens provides 10 percent of your daily value of calcium. The crunchy, tangy leaves of purslane are a good source of omega-3 fatty acids, vitamin C, and iron. Tight heads, such as romaine, radicchio, and Belgian endive, can be cut with a knife; all other greens should be torn. Include a variety of organic greens in your salads and you'll never get tired of eating them.

3. Always wash your greens. If they're beginning to wilt from sitting out too long, soak them in a large bowl or sink full of cold water. With greens such as spinach—where bits of dirt positively cling to the leaves—rinse two to three times to make sure all of the grit is washed away. If you don't use a produce wash, fill the sink with cold water and add four tablespoons of salt and some lemon juice. Soak greens for about ten minutes, then rinse them well. (It's important to wash nonorganic greens thoroughly to clean off as much of the pesticides as possible.)

When you get your greens and produce home from the market, wash them all at once and dry them thoroughly, then store everything in freezer zip-top bags to which you've added one or two white paper towels. This helps keep your produce fresh and makes it easy and fast to whip up your salads each day.

4. Make your own dressing, preferably just before serving the salad, but if you'd prefer to prepare a small batch, you can refrigerate it and use it up within a few days. Your dressing will only be as good as your ingredients, so purchase cold-pressed oils and keep them refrigerated. (The heat used to make commercial oils destroys many of the nutrients and causes the oil to break down more quickly, becoming rancid.) If you buy bottled dressings, see if there's an expiration date. Keep them refrigerated, too, and don't use condiments that have been in your refrigerator for months.

5. Don't overdress. Less is more when it comes to salad dressing. If you're using one that's higher in calories and want to cut back, keep it on the side and dip. After dressing the salad, toss well. The best instrument you can use is an impeccably clean pair of hands. I like to squeeze a bit of fresh lemon juice onto my salad, even over other dressings. It tastes great and makes the dressing go further. And don't forget, fresh lemon juice makes a simple, light, fat-free dressing for salads, too.

6. Create some finger salads. In a bowl, put a few crisp romaine leaves, a carrot, a couple stalks of celery, ½ sweet bell pepper, and whatever vegetables appeal to you—as close to the way nature made them as possible. Then simply use your hands instead of utensils and chew, chew, chew.

7. Use edible flowers. You can find edible flowers in many good produce markets. Also, refer to my book *Health Bliss* for more information. Experiment with different blossoms and their flavors. Creatively placing them around a plate or using them as a garnish can give an added touch of beauty to your meals. Of course, not all flowers are edible. Please don't pick your own unless you have a good guide and know exactly what you're doing.

8. Vary the amounts of the different ingredients, according to your taste. Think of salad recipes as guidelines, not a strict set of rules. They're here to help you get started on the road to vibrant heath.

VITALITY SALAD

You can't get much tastier than this simple, crispy salad. A great rejuvenator, alkalizer, and mild cleanser, this salad lends itself to any favorite occasion.
Serves 3–6.

2 cups romaine lettuce, torn into small pieces
1 cup baby spinach, stemmed
½ cup chopped celery
½ cup shredded carrot
½ cup shredded beet
½ cup diced jicama
½ cup diced ripe tomato
½ cup diced cucumber
¼ cup diced sweet pepper (red, yellow, or orange)
¼ cup sunflower seeds
Edible organic colorful flowers for garnish

In a bowl, combine all ingredients and toss with your favorite dressing.
Variations: Add beans, such as garbanzo or black beans; sunflower or pumpkin seeds; grilled tofu slices; or perhaps a scoop of quinoa or millet to make this salad a perfect, complete meal in a bowl.

SHREDDED RAINBOW SALAD

For your next large family gathering or party, make this salad in colorful layers in a large glass bowl, in individual Boston or butter-leaf lettuce cups, or on a bed of romaine lettuce on a beautiful platter. I guarantee it will be the hit of the party.
Serves 4.

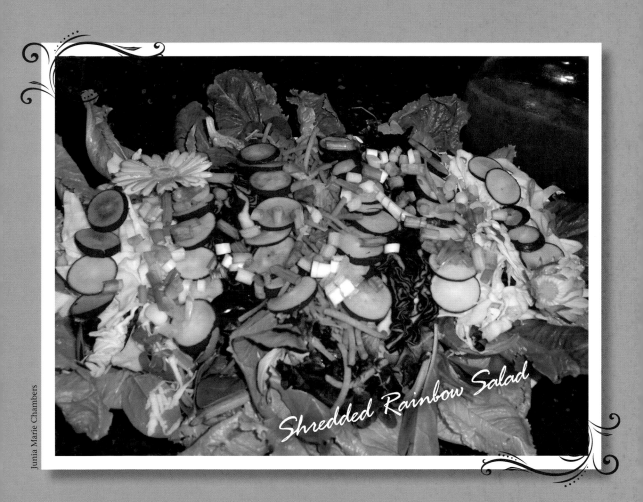

Shredded Rainbow Salad

Junia Marie Chambers

Tip: Wasabi and Pickled Ginger

Wasabi (Japanese horseradish) and pickled ginger are available in Asian markets and supermarkets with ample Asian-food sections. Wasabi is available in powdered form, which can be reconstituted with a few drops of water, or as a paste that comes in a small tube.

PEAR & ARUGULA SALAD WITH TOASTED WALNUTS

Arugula's delightful peppery flavor makes it one of my favorite leafy greens. Serves 2 as a main meal, 4–6 as a side salad.

2 small ripe Bartlett or Comice pears, cored and thinly sliced
7–8 oz. arugula
3 Tbsp. cold-pressed, extra-virgin olive oil
2 Tbsp. raspberry vinegar
⅛ tsp. sea salt
1 Tbsp. fresh chives, finely chopped
½ cup coarsely broken and toasted walnuts

Place the pears and arugula in a salad bowl. In a separate bowl, whisk together oil, vinegar, chives, and salt. Add the dressing to the pears and arugula and toss to combine. Toast the walnuts in a dry skillet over medium heat for 3–4 minutes, stirring constantly. Arrange salad on individual plates and sprinkle with the toasted walnuts.

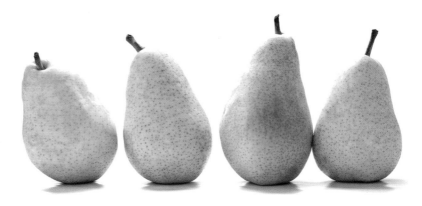

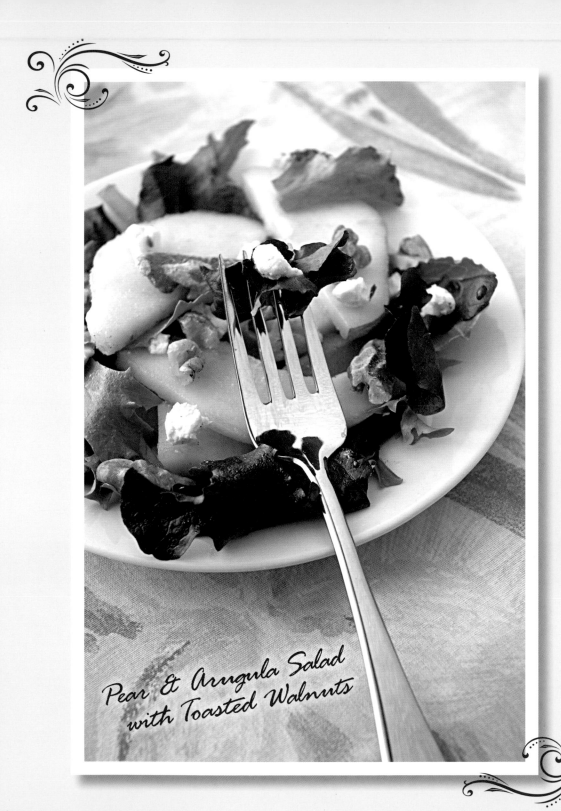

Pear & Arugula Salad
with Toasted Walnuts

CRUNCHY CABBAGE, APPLE & TURNIP SALAD WITH TOASTED CASHEWS

When I want something deliciously crunchy, this always hits the spot. Serves 4–6.

½ medium red cabbage, shredded
½ medium green cabbage, shredded
1 large apple, cored and chopped
1 small red onion, finely chopped
1 small turnip, grated
1 cup chopped fresh parsley
½ cup ground and toasted cashews

In a large bowl, combine all ingredients. Toss with a light vinaigrette to which you've added 1–2 Tbsp. fresh apple juice.

FYI: Turnips

Turnips are rich in calcium, magnesium, phosphorus, potassium, folic acid, and vitamin C. A very alkaline vegetable when eaten raw, turnips aid digestion and also help clear the blood of toxins.

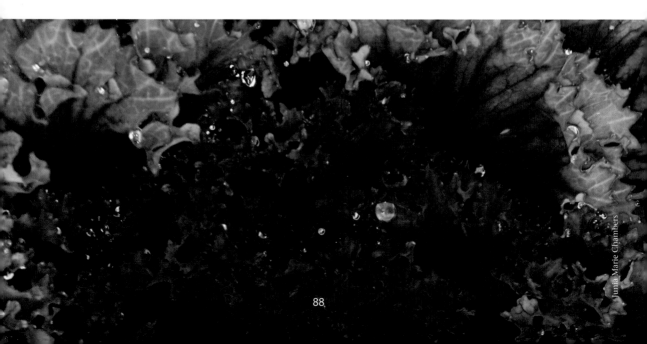

Junia Marie Chambers

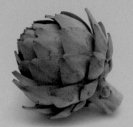
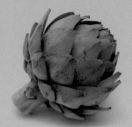
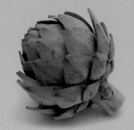

HEARTS OF ROMAINE, ARTICHOKE & PALM SALAD

This elegant simple salad always gets rave reviews.
Serves 4–6.

2 (9-oz.) packages frozen artichoke hearts, thawed, hearts cut in half
    (approx. 24 hearts)
1 can hearts of palm, drained and sliced ½-inch thick on an angle
¾ cup homemade vinaigrette (see Chapter 6)
3 Tbsp. chopped fresh parsley
1 clove garlic, minced
2 tsp. fresh lemon juice
3 romaine lettuce hearts, thoroughly washed and dried
2 sweet red or yellow bell peppers, roasted, peeled and sliced into thin strips
    (see Chapter 16)

In a bowl, combine artichoke hearts, hearts of palm, parsley, garlic, lemon juice, and dressing. Gently toss and chill. Now for the fun part: On individual salad plates, arrange the romaine hearts from the center out in a pinwheel design. With a slotted spoon, scoop the marinated hearts of palm and artichokes into the hub of the wheel. Then place the red and yellow roasted pepper strips in a crisscross pattern over the leaves and hearts. Drizzle some extra marinade dressing over the leaves and serve.

COUSCOUS GARDEN SALAD

I just love saying the word *couscous;* it makes me smile.

Serves 3–5.

¾ cup Vegetable Broth (see Chapter 7)
½ cup uncooked whole-grain couscous
¼ cup chopped green onion
¼ cup chopped yellow bell pepper
¼ cup chopped mushrooms
½ cup chopped Italian plum tomatoes
1 Tbsp. chopped fresh basil
1 tsp. chopped fresh tarragon
2 tsp. flaxseed oil or cold-pressed,
    extra-virgin olive oil
1 tsp. fresh lemon juice
1 tsp. organic balsamic vinegar
2 cups baby spinach or 1 head of Bibb or
    butter lettuce
⅓ cup ground and toasted cashews, for garnish
3–5 lemon slices, for garnish

In a saucepan, bring broth to a boil. Remove from heat and stir in couscous. Cover and let stand until cool, then fluff with a fork. In a separate mixing bowl, combine vegetables, tomatoes, herbs, oil, lemon juice, and vinegar. Mix well. Add the couscous and combine thoroughly. Cover and refrigerate for about 1 hour or until chilled. Serve on a bed of baby spinach or large leaves of Bibb lettuce. Garnish with lemon slices and sprinkle with ground, toasted cashews.

Variation: Before stirring the couscous into the broth to steam it, dry sauté ¼ cup of the couscous in a skillet for about 2–3 minutes. It will turn a darker shade and become imbued with a nuttier flavor. (I usually toast only half so that the nutty flavor doesn't overwhelm the salad.) Cook both the toasted and remaining dry couscous together and proceed with the recipe.

Tip: Couscous

A delectable, easy-to-digest, grain-based food, couscous is feather-light and fluffy and cooks up in minutes. Traditional in North Africa, couscous is made from the endosperm of durum wheat (and therefore must be avoided by anyone with a gluten allergy). It's delicious as pilaf, or enjoy it as a dessert by baking with apple juice and your favorite fruits and nuts.

APRICOT-SPINACH SALAD

This can be enjoyed as a side salad or a marvelous main course. How you use it determines the number of servings it yields.

Serves 2–6.

4 cups baby spinach, washed and dried
½ cup chopped dried apricots (unsulfured)
⅓ cup chopped green onions
⅓ cup diced yellow bell pepper
3 Tbsp. toasted sunflower seeds
1 Tbsp. toasted sesame seeds
4 Tbsp. plain, nondairy yogurt
2 Tbsp. organic balsamic vinegar
2 Tbsp. fresh orange juice
1 Tbsp. fresh lemon juice
1 tsp. orange zest (from an organic orange only)
1 clove garlic

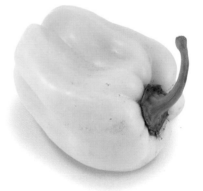

In a large bowl, toss the spinach, apricots, green onion, bell pepper, and sunflower and sesame seeds. In a separate bowl, combine the remaining ingredients. Pour over the salad and toss to combine. Serve right away, or chill for about one hour.

Variation: Substitute currants, raisins, or dried cherries for the apricots.

FYI: Spinach

Spinach is rich in beta-carotene, potassium, iron, vitamin B_6, vitamin C, calcium, and magnesium. It helps fight cancer, heart disease, and mental disorders due to its high folic-acid content. An excellent antioxidant, it helps regulate blood pressure and boosts the immune system. It's an excellent anticancer food, supports bone density, and has the ability to rev up your metabolism and accelerate fat loss. Spinach has only 6 calories per ½ cup when eaten raw and 20 calories when cooked. It's definitely worth making this antioxidant superfood a mainstay of your diet.

SOBA-NOODLE SALAD WITH GARDEN VEGETABLES

Soba—a thin, delicious, high-protein Japanese-style pasta—is often served in a broth or chilled and served with a dipping sauce. Look for either organic whole-wheat or buckwheat (my favorite) soba at your natural-food store or Asian market.

Serves 4–6.

12 oz. soba noodles
1 cup broccoli florets
1 cup cauliflower pieces
2 carrots, peeled and cut on an angle into ¼-inch slices
¾ cup sliced water chestnuts
3 green onions, chopped
¾ cup sliced bamboo shoots, drained
½–1 cup vinaigrette (see Chapter 6),
    depending on your taste buds—less is more for me
2 Tbsp. toasted sesame seeds

Cook soba noodles according to the package directions, drain, and chill. Lightly steam the broccoli, cauliflower, and carrots. Chill. In a large bowl, combine the chilled noodles, the chilled vegetables, chestnuts, green onions, bamboo shoots, and dressing of your choice. Refrigerate for at least one hour before serving, mixing occasionally so the flavors blend. Garnish with toasted sesame seeds.

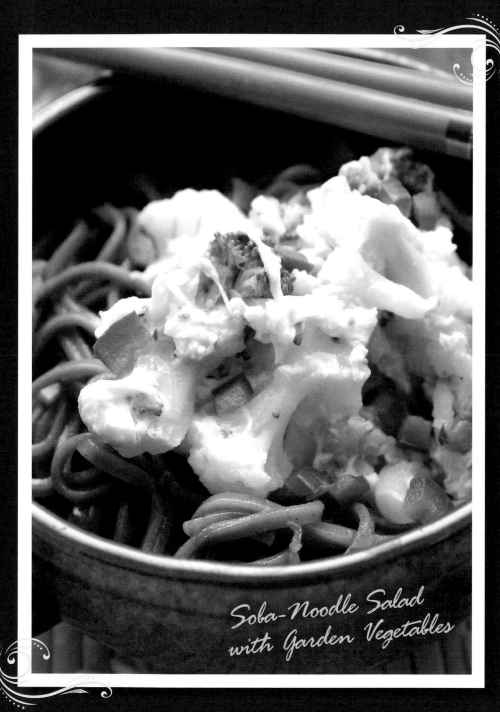

Soba-Noodle Salad
with Garden Vegetables

PARSLEY-LENTIL SALAD

For color, taste, and an abundance of nutrients, this salad is hard to beat. It's also delicious scooped into warm, whole-grain pita triangles.
Serves 4–6.

1½ cups dry lentils (about 10 oz.)
2 cups Vegetable Broth (see Chapter 7)
1 bay leaf
2 red peppers, roasted and cut into ½-inch pieces (see Chapter 16)
1 small red onion, thinly sliced
2 medium organic lemons
1½ cups loosely packed, fresh parsley leaves, finely chopped
¼ cup cold-pressed, extra-virgin olive oil
1 tsp. Bragg Liquid Aminos, low-sodium tamari, or shoyu
¼ tsp. fresh coarsely ground black pepper
⅛ tsp. garlic powder

Rinse lentils well with cold running water; discard any stones or blemished lentils. In a large saucepan, place lentils, bay leaf, and enough water or Vegetable Broth to cover lentils by 2 inches. Bring to a boil; reduce to simmer and cover. Cook for 20 minutes or until lentils are tender. Discard bay leaf. Place the sliced onion in a colander and drain lentils over the onion to soften it just a bit and take away its strong bite. Grate 2 teaspoons lemon peel (zest) and squeeze ¼ cup lemon juice. In a big mixing bowl, combine lentils, roasted peppers, parsley, lemon juice and peel, oil, garlic powder, Bragg Liquid Aminos (or alternative), and pepper. Serve warm or chilled.

FYI: Lentils

Lentils are an excellent source of protein, calcium, magnesium, phosphorus, potassium, zinc, and folic acid. These nutrients benefit nearly every organ and system in the body. The organic green lentil is the classic one to use for soups as it "melts" in just 30 minutes, making a thick, smooth base to which you can add all your favorite vegetables and seasonings. The Beluga are tiny black lentils indigenous to Syria; they look like caviar and are heavenly. They're higher in protein than French, green, or red varieties. Try them in salads or soups. French lentils, actually a Persian variety, are tiny gray to green-black ovals. Crimson (red) lentils are famous for their beauty and flavor, and they bring elegance to any dish. Always buy organic lentils.

SPICY BLACK-BEAN SALAD

This high-protein dish is great as a snack, side dish, or main meal.
Serves 4–6.

3 cups cooked, chilled black beans
1 red or yellow bell pepper, diced
1 large carrot, diced
2 Tbsp. chopped fresh cilantro
½ fresh lemon, juiced
Dash ground cumin
Dash cayenne pepper or crushed red-pepper flakes
Sea salt to taste

Combine everything in a large bowl and serve at room temperature on a bed of crisp lettuce leaves.

Variation: Substitute another type of bean, such as navy, garbanzo, pinto, black-eyed, Anasazi, lima, butterscotch, calypso, azuki (aduki), kidney, or a combination.

Tip: Cooking Beans

Being concentrated sources of protein, beans need to be soaked for at least 4 hours before cooking, preferably overnight. If you forget, there's a quick-soak method: Bring beans to a boil, then let sit for one hour. Soaking beans overnight and/or cooking with kombu (a sea vegetable) enhances their digestibility. After soaking, always pour the water out and add fresh water for cooking. Also, if you're going to add salt, don't put it in until the beans have finished cooking because salt toughens the beans' skins.

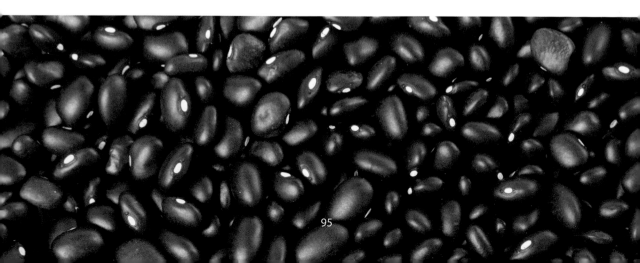

CUCUMBER-TOFU SALAD WITH TOASTED PECANS

This low-calorie, high-protein salad is elegant enough for the most discriminating party guests and easy enough to whip up at the last minute.

Serves 4–6.

1 (12.3-oz.) package extra-firm organic silken tofu
5–6 large celery stalks, juiced (¾ cup)
1 small lemon, juiced
1 Tbsp. white or yellow miso
¼ tsp. sea salt
7 radishes, thinly sliced
4 large cucumbers, thinly sliced (peeled, if not organic)
4 green onions, finely chopped
¼ cup finely chopped fresh parsley
¼ cup finely chopped fresh mint
½ cup pecans, toasted (dry sauté 4–5 minutes in a skillet), for garnish

In a food processor or blender, combine the lemon juice, celery juice, tofu, miso, and salt until creamy smooth. In a large salad bowl, combine the rest of the ingredients, except the pecans, with the dressing. Chill for at least one hour. Arrange the salad on individual plates or on a bed of crisp greens and garnish with toasted pecans.

Variation: Instead of pecans, substitute toasted coarsely ground almonds, cashews, pine nuts, or sesame seeds.

FYI: Cucumbers

Cucumbers are a dieter's best friend since they're very low in calories and rich in potassium and beta-carotene. They're naturally diuretic and laxative and dissolve the uric acid that causes kidney and bladder stones. They support digestion and regulate blood pressure.

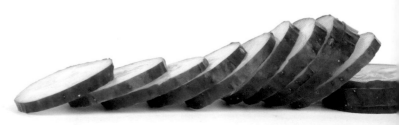

FOUR-BEAN SALAD

This tastes best with fresh-cut beans, but if you only have canned or frozen, they'll work just fine.
Serves 4–6.

½ lb. fresh green beans, trimmed and cut into 1½-inch pieces
    (or 8-oz. canned)
½ lb. fresh wax beans, trimmed and cut into 1½-inch pieces (or 8-oz. canned)
1 cup cooked kidney beans (or 8-oz. canned)
1 cup cooked garbanzo beans (chickpeas) (or 8-oz. canned)
1 8-oz. can sliced water chestnuts
1 medium red onion, cut into ½-inch dice
½ cup sliced green onion
1 yellow pepper, cut into ½-inch dice

If using fresh beans, steam trimmed beans in a stockpot about 7–8 minutes (you want them to be slightly crunchy/slightly tender). Transfer beans to a large bowl. Add the rest of the ingredients and combine thoroughly. Chill, then toss with the dressing of your choice.
Variation: Substitute asparagus or broccoli for the green beans. If you use all canned beans, just make sure to rinse and drain the beans first. This makes them less gas-producing and reduces the sodium. You can also buy canned beans without sodium.

SUNNY SHREDDED-DILL & TOASTED-SESAME COLESLAW

This easy-to-make salad provides lots of fiber with very few calories.
Serves 6–8.

2 cups shredded red cabbage
2 cups shredded green cabbage
2 carrots, peeled and grated
1 small daikon, peeled and grated
3 stalks bok choy, white parts only, cut into ⅛-inch slices

2 Tbsp. toasted sesame seeds
1 Tbsp. dill seeds

In a large bowl, combine all ingredients and toss with the dressing of your choice. I like to use Lemon Tahini dressing (see Chapter 6).

Variation: To add more minerals and variety to this coleslaw, I like to include a package of wakame, a large, brown sea vegetable (seaweed). Just soak wakame in scalding water for 15 minutes, then strain. With the tip of a sharp knife, remove the thick membrane and julienne ¼-inch pieces from the outer leaves. Toss with the rest of the ingredients.

FYI: Cabbage

Long a staple in Eastern Europe, cabbage is versatile, tasty, filling, and loaded with effective anticancer and antioxidant agents. Drinking cabbage juice is very beneficial for ulcers. If you've only eaten red or green cabbage, it's time to branch out. Look for savoy, or Chinese cabbage, an elongated bundle of leaves with a core; and bok choy, another Asian cabbage with plump white stalks and green floppy leaves.

FYI: Daikon

Daikon contains the digestive enzymes diastase, amylase, and esterase, and contains a substance that inhibits the formation of carcinogens in the body. If you've never tried this easy-to-grow Japanese radish, rush to the nearest store. It's a pearly white root that's shaped like a carrot and can grow as long as your arm. You don't even need to peel it. Just wash and grate it to use raw in a salad, to garnish grains, or to use (as you would use a carrot) in soups or sautéed, simmered, baked, or braised dishes.

COLORFUL SUMMER-FRUIT COMBO

For breakfast, a midmorning or midafternoon snack, or a light lunch or dinner, this fresh-fruit combo combines the most luscious colors and flavors for a delightful treat. Be creative! Almost any fruit will work in this salad.

Serves 2–6.

1 small or ½ medium cantaloupe, sliced and cubed
½ medium honeydew melon, sliced and cubed
2 pears, peeled and cubed
2 cups sweet cherries, pitted
1 cup berries of your choice

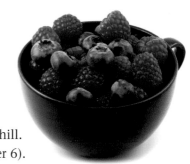

In a large bowl, combine all of the ingredients and chill. If desired, top with one of my fruit dressings (see Chapter 6).

FYI: Cherries

Sweet cherries have only 50 calories per ½ cup (uncooked). They have a natural laxative effect and are an excellent component of an elimination or detox diet. Being high in iron, they're a natural blood builder. A one-cup serving supplies almost 25 percent of the RDA of vitamin A, along with a moderate amount of fiber. And like most fruits and vegetables, they're virtually free of sodium and fat. For a sweet-tooth craving, these usually hit the spot. Keep organic frozen dark sweet cherries on hand to sweeten your smoothies.

ANTIOXIDANT-RICH SPINACH & SWEET-POTATO SALAD

The colors and sweetness in this salad appeal to children and teens as well as adults. When I make this as my entire meal, I sometimes add beans or tofu, grilled or sautéed and cut into strips, or a few nuts and seeds to increase the protein.
Serves 2–6.

4 cups baby spinach, washed and stemmed
1 small red pepper, diced
1 small yellow pepper, diced
2 cups sweet potatoes, peeled, diced, and steamed; warm or chilled

In a large bowl, combine all ingredients and dress with Orange Balsamic Vinaigrette, Orange Sesame-Cashew Dressing, or Orange Sweet-Potato Dressing (see Chapter 6).

FYI: Sweet Potatoes

Another superfood, sweet potatoes are a root vegetable, not a tuber like white potatoes. They provide calcium, magnesium, potassium, folic acid, vitamins C and E, phosphorus, and loads of beta-carotene. Easily digestible and highly nutritious, they're excellent for inflammation of the digestive tract, ulcers, and poor circulation. They're also detoxifying as they bind to heavy metals to help remove them from the body. The National Cancer Institute has indicated that eating ½ cup per day of sweet potatoes or other bright orange vegetables, such as carrots and winter squash, can cut the likelihood of lung cancer by as much as 50 percent.

SUN-DRIED TOMATO, HIJIKI & ROMAINE SALAD

This very low-calorie, mineral-rich salad will fill you up and boost your energy.

Serves 2–6.

2 cups romaine lettuce hearts, torn into bite-size pieces

1½ cups combination of arugula and baby spinach, torn into bite-size pieces

½ cup cucumber, peeled, seeded, and chopped

½ cup grated daikon

½ cup chopped sweet yellow, orange, or purple bell peppers

6–8 sun-dried tomatoes (not the ones packed in oil), soaked in water, drained, and chopped

3 Tbsp. green onions, finely chopped

1½ Tbsp. dried hijiki, soaked in water for 30 minutes, drained and chopped

Fresh parsley sprigs, for garnish

In a large bowl, combine the lettuce and spinach leaves with the cucumber, daikon, bell peppers, tomatoes, green onions, and hijiki. Toss the salad with Grapefruit Mustard Dressing (see Chapter 6). Garnish with fresh parsley sprigs and serve.

FYI: Hijiki (Hiziki)

This low-calorie seaweed is the most mineral-rich of all of the sea vegetables. It looks like long, narrow, black ribbons. It grows near the low-water mark along the Japanese coast and is harvested in the winter and spring, after which it's sun-dried, boiled, and dried again. Its slightly salty flavor and cooling action make it a superior kidney food. It also acts as a diuretic, detoxifies the body, supports the thyroid and bones, and stabilizes blood sugar. One cup of cooked hijiki contains more calcium than a cup of milk. It's also a rich source of iron, protein, vitamin A, and B vitamins.

JICAMA-LEEK & PEPPER SALAD

I love the crunchy sweetness of jicama in salads, as part of a raw vegetable or fruit plate, or diced in grains and casseroles.

Serves 4–6.

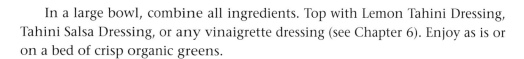

2 cups diced jicama
2 leeks, finely diced
1 red bell pepper, diced
1 yellow bell pepper, diced
1 large avocado, peeled and diced
1 jalapeno pepper, seeds and white ribs removed, diced (optional)
2 green onions, finely diced
2 stalks celery, finely diced

In a large bowl, combine all ingredients. Top with Lemon Tahini Dressing, Tahini Salsa Dressing, or any vinaigrette dressing (see Chapter 6). Enjoy as is or on a bed of crisp organic greens.

FYI: Leeks

Leeks are an excellent source of fiber, potassium, vitamins K and A, calcium, folic acid, and the lesser-known carotenoids lutein and zeaxanthin. Leeks are cleansing and diuretic, and they can help eliminate uric acid in gout.

Tip: Leeks

A sweet cousin of the onion, the leek is a versatile root vegetable that's great in salads, soups, sautéed dishes, pilafs, and casseroles. Many recipes call for cutting off the green tops and only using the white part, but I disagree. I use not only the leek's green leaf but also its many tiny rootlets, which are mineral-dense filaments that add valuable flavor and nutrients. The only parts to discard are the dehydrated end and any large, tough outer leaves. Slice the remaining vegetable in half lengthwise and wash very carefully, making sure to remove any dirt lodged in the leaves.

Tip: Jicama

Pronounced "HICK-uh-muh," this root vegetable looks like a beige, oversize turnip. Peel it and you'll find crisp, slightly sweet flesh that's similar to water chestnuts—only crunchier. Very low in calories, it's a good source of potassium. Jicama is a nice addition to any vegetable tray because its neutral flavor lends itself well to most dips.

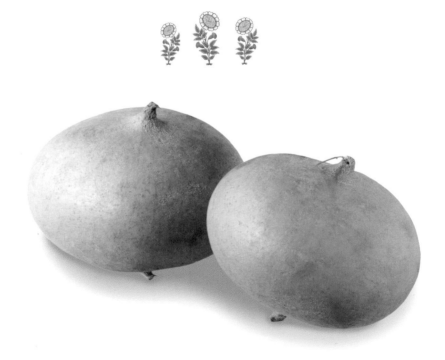

CHAPTER 6

DRESSINGS & TOPPINGS

*"I submit that scientists have not yet explored the
hidden possibilities of the innumerable seeds, leaves,
and fruit for giving the fullest possible nutrition to mankind."*

— MAHATMA GANDHI

Many people make the mistake of preparing a healthful salad and then drowning it with an artery-clogging, high-fat dressing. When you use dressings on a salad, don't make the mistake of pouring on so much that you can hardly taste the vegetables. Less is always more when it comes to these condiments. In addition to enhancing salads, I use many of these dressings over steamed vegetables or grains and as dips for raw vegetables or artichoke leaves.

Remember, instead of always using a dressing, you can drizzle some fresh lemon juice over your salad, or even combine fresh grapefruit juice with a couple of drops of tamari or Bragg Liquid Aminos. Fresh dressing is so much better tasting and better for you than bottled ones. Get in the habit of making yours fresh and using them within three days. Look for the freshest cold-pressed oils, such as extra-virgin olive, which is the best next to an organic, cold-pressed flaxseed or hemp oil. (I use hemp oil by Living Harvest.) Also try a variety of vinegars, such as organic balsamic raspberry, brown rice, raw apple cider, fig, and red wine.

You'll be surprised by how quickly and easily you can make delicious dressings right in your own kitchen, where you can totally control the ingredients and create the exact tastes that you love.

Fat-Free Dressings on the Run

When you don't have time to make your dressing from scratch, check out your natural-food store and see what you can find that appeals to you in the nonfat and low-fat categories. (Be sure to check the label on the *back* of the bottle. The front is frequently misleading.) While healthful bottled dressings aren't as fresh as homemade, they're head and shoulders above conventional offerings. They also double as excellent marinades on grilled vegetables.

Have you ever used a marinara or other pasta sauce as a salad dressing? It's different and quick. Make sure you get fat-free, low-sodium varieties. Besides the great taste of tomato-based sauces, you get an extra helping of lycopene, the phytonutrient that may help reduce the risk of cancer and heart disease. Another easy way to save time is to modify one of the creations you've already made from the recipes in Chapter 4. Usually, you can just add a little liquid to thin a spread, sauce, or dip.

VITALITY VINAIGRETTE

This easy, healthful, and delicious vinaigrette is my favorite dressing, the one that I make more than any other.

Makes about ¾ cup.

⅓ cup fresh lemon juice (juice of 2 medium lemons)
2 Tbsp. organic balsamic vinegar
1 tsp. garlic, pressed (2–3 cloves)
1 tsp. Dijon mustard
⅛ tsp. sea salt
⅓ cup flaxseed oil (or hemp oil or cold-pressed, extra-virgin olive oil)

Whisk together the lemon juice, vinegar, garlic, mustard, and salt until well blended. Drizzle in a little oil at a time, whisking after each addition until all of the oil is thoroughly incorporated. Use within 3 days.

Variations: You can substitute other vinegars, such as raw apple-cider, raspberry, brown-rice, red-wine, or peach vinegar, either for half or all of the balsamic vinegar.

Tip: Juicing a Lemon

To get the most juice from a lemon, roll it back and forth on a hard counter for a few seconds, then cut it open and squeeze. I use a wooden citrus reamer daily and wouldn't be without it in my healthy kitchen.

VITALITY FRENCH VINAIGRETTE

Everyone raves about this dressing.
Makes 2 cups.

¾ cup basic Vitality Vinaigrette (see preceding recipe)
1 large ripe tomato, cut into quarters

Blend all ingredients in a blender or food processor on high speed for 30 seconds. Use within 3 days.

Variations: Add 1–2 tsp. each of any of the following chopped or minced fresh herbs: basil, chervil, chives, cilantro, dill, herbes de Provence, lemongrass, mint, oregano, parsley, rosemary, tarragon, or thyme.

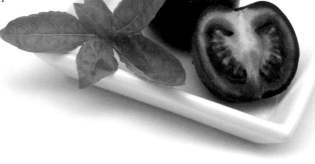

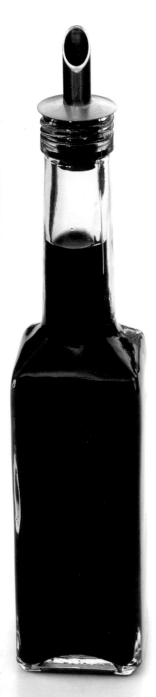

VITALITY THOUSAND ISLAND

This dressing is light, colorful, and refreshing on any salad with crisp greens. Try it as a topping on grains, potatoes, and steamed vegetables, as well as over tofu steaks and on soba or other whole-grain pasta/noodles.
Makes 2½ cups.

2 cups Vitality French Vinaigrette (see preceding recipe)
6 oz. extra-firm lite organic silken tofu or nondairy yogurt

In a blender or food processor, blend vinaigrette and tofu at high speed for 30 seconds. Use within 3 days.

NEVER-FAIL HERB VINAIGRETTE

This one is quick and easy—great on any green salad or sprinkled over lightly steamed or roasted veggies.
Makes about ¾ cup.

¼ cup red-wine vinegar
1 Tbsp. finely chopped fresh parsley leaves
1 Tbsp. finely chopped fresh chives
1 tsp. finely chopped fresh tarragon leaves
1 tsp. finely chopped fresh chervil
½ tsp. sea salt
¼ tsp. coarsely ground fresh black pepper
½ cup cold-pressed, extra-virgin olive oil

In a small bowl, whisk together all ingredients except the oil until thoroughly blended. Whisk in the oil a little at a time. Cover and refrigerate for up to 3 days if not using right away.
Variations: Substitute organic balsamic vinegar for the red-wine vinegar. For garlic vinaigrette: Add 2–3 medium garlic cloves, finely minced. For lemon vinaigrette: Substitute fresh lemon juice for the red-wine vinegar. For Dijon vinaigrette: Add 1 Tbsp. Dijon mustard.

EASY BALSAMIC-DIJON VINAIGRETTE FOR TWO

With this simple recipe, you'll never want to resort to bottled dressings again.

Makes about ⅓ cup.

1–2 Tbsp. cold-pressed, extra-virgin olive oil (I use only 1 Tbsp.)
2 Tbsp. organic balsamic vinegar
1 medium clove garlic, minced
¼ tsp. Dijon mustard
⅛ tsp. sea salt
⅛ tsp. coarsely ground fresh black pepper

In a small jar with a tight-fitting lid, combine all ingredients and shake until thoroughly incorporated or blended. Pour over salad of your choice and toss to coat. Use within 3 days.

ORANGE-BALSAMIC VINAIGRETTE

Your taste buds will adore this wonderful vinaigrette variation.

Makes about ½ cup.

3 Tbsp. cold-pressed, extra-virgin olive oil
1 Tbsp. fresh orange juice
1 Tbsp. organic balsamic vinegar
1 tsp. honey Dijon mustard (or regular Dijon sweetened with agave nectar or
    brown-rice syrup, if you want to avoid honey)
1 tsp. orange zest (from an organic orange only)
¼ tsp. sea salt

In a jar or small bowl, thoroughly combine all ingredients. Just before serving, drizzle over your salad and toss. Use within 3 days.

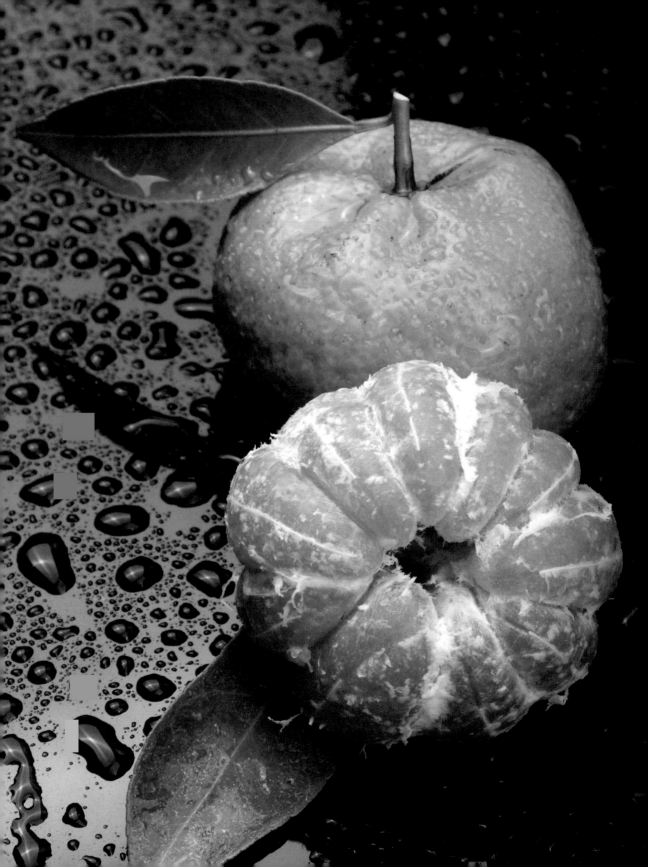

TANGERINE-UME DRESSING

This refreshing and unusual dressing is great tossed on your favorite vegetable or noodle salad. Umeboshi plums are available fresh or in paste form in natural- and Asian-food stores.

Makes about ½ cup.

Juice of 2 medium tangerines
3 Tbsp. raw tahini
1 Tbsp. cold-pressed sesame oil
1 Tbsp. purified water
1 Tbsp. fresh lemon juice
2 tsp. umeboshi paste or minced umeboshi (pickled Japanese plums)
1 clove garlic, minced
1 tsp. chives, for garnish

In a blender or food processor, blend all ingredients except the chives until smooth. Add the chives and chill for 30 minutes before using. Use within 3 days.

Variation: Substitute fresh orange or grapefruit juice for the tangerine juice. If using grapefruit juice, add 2 teaspoons brown-rice syrup to sweeten the dressing.

LEMON-MUSTARD DRESSING

One of my all-time favorites. I often give this dressing as a gift in a beautiful glass jar, garnished with a pretty ribbon on top.

Makes about 2½ cups.

6 oz. firm lite organic silken tofu
½ cup plain or lemon nondairy yogurt or Lemonaise Spread (see Chapter 4)
¼ cup purified water
¼ cup fresh lemon juice (omit if using lemon nondairy yogurt
    or Lemonaise Spread)
¼ cup brown-rice vinegar
¼ cup stone-ground mustard, low-sodium
2–3 cloves garlic, minced

1 Tbsp. chopped fresh Italian parsley
1 Tbsp. chopped fresh tarragon
1–2 tsp. minced red onion
¼ tsp. sea salt
Dash cayenne pepper

Thoroughly blend all ingredients in a blender or food processor.

ORANGE SESAME-CASHEW DRESSING

On a crisp romaine or baby-spinach salad with cucumber, hearts of palm, and red bell pepper, nothing tastes better.

Makes about ¾ cup.

¼ cup unhulled sesame seeds
10 raw cashews
2 Tbsp. mango, peach, raspberry, or
    other fruit vinegar
3 medium oranges, peeled and diced (or
    3 tangerines or 1 jar of unsweetened
    mandarin-orange slices)
½ cup fresh orange juice
⅛ tsp. sea salt

Toast the sesame seeds in a dry, hot skillet for 3–4 minutes, stirring occasionally so they don't burn. In a blender or food processor, blend together the orange juice, ¼ cup orange pieces, cashews, vinegar, and 2 tablespoons of roasted sesame seeds. Next, add the remaining orange pieces to the salad and toss with the dressing. Sprinkle the extra toasted sesame seeds on the top. Use right away.

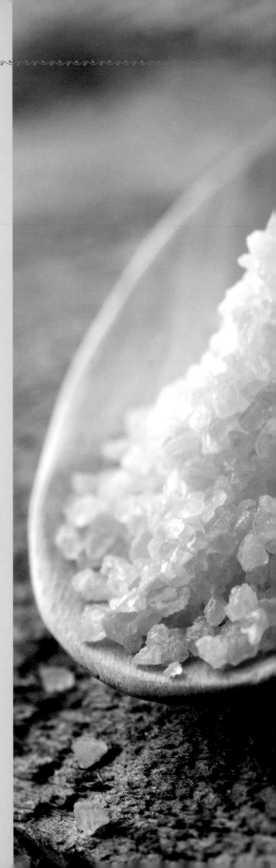

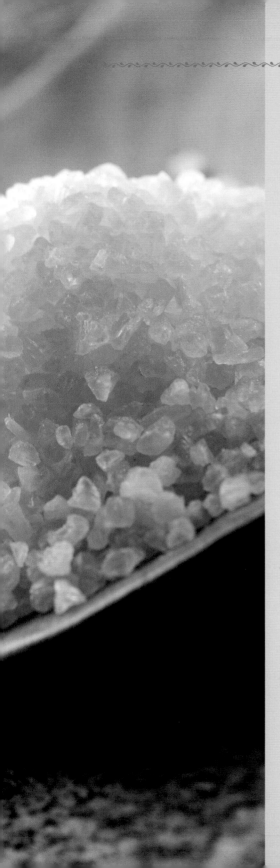

CILANTRO THOUSAND ISLAND

This is a healthful, low-fat version of thousand-island dressing for cilantro lovers everywhere.

Makes about 2¾ cups.

⅓ cup diced red bell pepper
2 Tbsp. chopped fresh cilantro
¼ cup diced onion
1 Tbsp. chopped green olives
1 Tbsp. chopped fresh Italian parsley
4 oz. firm lite organic silken tofu, cut into 1½-inch cubes (or 4 oz. nondairy yogurt)
⅔ cup organic tomato purée
½ cup purified water
½ cup plain nondairy yogurt (in addition to the above if you didn't use tofu)
¼ cup brown-rice syrup
⅛ tsp. sea salt

In a food processor, combine red pepper, cilantro, olives, onion, and parsley. Set aside. In a blender, purée the remaining ingredients. Add the puréed mixture to the food processor and pulse until desired consistency. If you want to make it creamier, blend on high speed for 15–20 seconds. Use within 5 days. Keep refrigerated.

DILL HONEY-MUSTARD

This is great on salads and steamed vegetables, especially broccoli or cauliflower florets.

Makes about ¾ cup.

½ cup plain nondairy yogurt
¼ cup purified water
1 Tbsp. honey Dijon mustard (or regular Dijon sweetened with agave nectar or
    brown-rice syrup, if you want to avoid honey)
1 Tbsp. white miso
2 tsp. dried dill or 1 ½ Tbsp. minced fresh dill
Dash or two of hot sauce

In a small bowl, combine all ingredients and whisk to blend. Use within 5 days. Keep refrigerated.

LEMON TAHINI

This is another one of my favorite dressings that's a rich source of protein, calcium, and omega-3s.
Makes about ½ cup.

⅓ cup purified water
¼ cup raw or roasted tahini (pour off any oil that has risen to the top of the jar)
2 Tbsp. fresh squeezed lemon juice
Sea salt to taste

Blend all ingredients in a blender or food processor until smooth. Add more water if you prefer a thinner consistency. Use within 5 days. Keep refrigerated.
Variation: Add some minced garlic, chopped parsley, or a dash of cumin or turmeric and blend.

DELUXE TAHINI

If you like tahini, you'll love this recipe. It's worth the extra preparation time.
Makes about 2 cups.

1½ cups warm water
8 oz. raw or roasted tahini

3 cloves garlic, minced
Juice of one large lemon
1 tsp. low-sodium tamari or Bragg Liquid Aminos
2 Tbsp. chopped fresh parsley
2 tsp. raw apple-cider vinegar
1 tsp. dried basil
½ tsp. ground coriander
¼ tsp. ground cumin
3–4 dashes Tabasco sauce
Pinch freshly ground pepper
1 tsp. sea salt (optional)

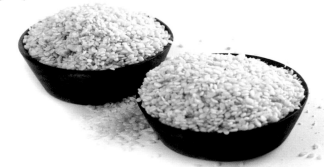

Blend all ingredients in a blender or food processor until smooth. Store in a covered jar in the refrigerator. Use within 6 days.

FYI: Tahini

Tahini is hulled sesame-seed paste, and while it's comparatively high in fat, its nutritional and culinary virtues warrant its inclusion in a healthful diet. It's high in calcium, omega-3s, iron, zinc, magnesium, vitamin E, and folic acid; and it's the perfect creamy ingredient for salad dressings, soups, and sauces. Because of its higher caloric content, don't overdo consumption if losing weight is your goal. Enjoying it a few times weekly in small amounts is okay.

TAHINI-SALSA DRESSING

This gives any salad a Tex-Mex flavor and turns the basic tahini dressing into a lower-calorie, lycopene-rich topping. It's also great as a sauce on potatoes and steamed vegetables and as a dip for raw vegetables.

Makes about 2 cups.

1 cup Lemon Tahini or Deluxe Tahini (see preceding recipes)
1 cup Sensational Salsa (see Chapter 4)

In a medium bowl, combine the dressing and the salsa thoroughly and serve. Store in the refrigerator for up to 5 days.

TAHINI-MINT DRESSING

This refreshing version of tahini dressing is heavenly—toss with chickpeas, carrots, diced cucumbers, and red onions on a bed of Boston or romaine lettuce or stuff into whole-grain pita bread.

Makes about ¾ cup.

1 cup loosely packed, chopped fresh mint leaves
¼ cup raw tahini
¼ cup purified water
3 Tbsp. fresh lemon juice
½ tsp. lemon zest (from an organic lemon only)
⅛ tsp. low-sodium tamari

Blend all ingredients in a blender or food processor until smooth. Store in the refrigerator. Use within 5 days.

ORANGE SWEET-POTATO DRESSING

This beta-carotene-rich dressing adds distinctive flavor and color to any salad. Try it on grilled vegetables, too.

Makes about 1¾ cups.

½ cup steamed sweet potato
½ cup fresh orange juice
2 Tbsp. cold-pressed, extra-virgin olive oil
1 Tbsp. organic balsamic vinegar
2 tsp. lemon juice
2 tsp. white or yellow miso
1 tsp. orange zest (from an organic orange only)
1 tsp. nutritional yeast
Dash cayenne pepper

Steam yam until soft. Cool, peel, and cut into 1½-inch pieces. Combine all ingredients in a blender or food processor and blend until smooth. Keep in the refrigerator. Use within 5 days.

GINGER-PEAR VINAIGRETTE

The combination of pear and ginger together make this dressing a heavenly treat—especially tossed with Hearts of Romaine, Artichoke & Palm Salad (see Chapter 5).
Makes about ½ cup.

1 pear
2 Tbsp. fresh lemon juice
⅛-inch slice of ginger, juiced
¼ cup cold-pressed walnut or sesame oil
2 Tbsp. brown rice or balsamic vinegar
Sea salt to taste

Juice the pear and ginger together. Then in a small bowl, whisk together the pear-ginger juice with the remaining ingredients. Use within 3 days.

ZESTY AVOCADO DRESSING

If you're looking for a terrific topping for your baked potatoes so that you won't miss butter and sour cream, this one is perfect.
Makes about 1½ cups.

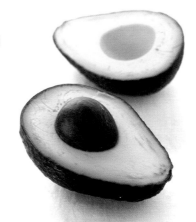

1 ripe avocado, peeled, pitted, and sliced
½ tomato, diced
½ cup celery juice or water
¼ cup plain nondairy yogurt
1 clove garlic, minced or pressed
1 Tbsp. finely chopped fresh tarragon
2 tsp. fresh lemon juice
4 basil leaves
Dash sea salt
Dash cayenne pepper

Blend all ingredients in a blender or food processor until smooth. Keep in the refrigerator. Use within 2 days.

SPICY CASHEW DRESSING

For topping udon or soba noodles, whether cold or warm, this spicy dressing will work well.

Makes 3–4 cups.

1 cup unsalted cashew butter (available at natural-food stores)
2–3 cups water, depending on the consistency you want
2 cloves garlic, pressed
1 Tbsp. fresh ginger, grated
2 tsp. white or yellow miso
½ tsp. cayenne pepper, to taste

Blend all ingredients in a blender or food processor until smooth. Keep in the refrigerator. Use within 4 days.

Variations: Substitute natural, unsalted peanut butter or almond butter for the cashew butter.

MISO-WALNUT-BASIL DRESSING/TOPPING

Besides using this recipe as an elegant dressing for salads, try it on top of vegetables or potatoes.

Makes about 2½ cups.

1¼ cups plain nondairy yogurt
1 cup walnuts
1 Tbsp. amber-colored miso
1½ tsp. fresh lemon juice
½ tsp. brown-rice vinegar
8 basil leaves

Roast the walnuts in a large, heavy skillet over medium heat, stirring constantly, for 5–6 minutes. Blend all ingredients in a blender or food processor until chunky. Use within 3 days.

FABULOUS FRUIT DRESSING/TOPPING

Using this topping over chilled fresh fruit makes a delicious, nutritious breakfast. Top with ground almonds or walnuts to make it a complete, balanced meal.
Makes about 3 cups.

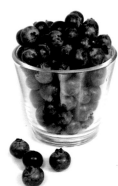

½ cup pineapple chunks
½ cup blueberries
½ cup strawberries
½ cup seedless grapes
1 ripe banana
¼ cup fresh apple juice
¼ cup fresh orange juice
⅛ tsp. cinnamon

Blend all ingredients in a blender or food processor until smooth. Chill in the refrigerator before serving. Pour over fresh fruit of your choice. Use within 2 days.

Variations: Triple the recipe and pour the blended fruit mixture into ice-cube trays and freeze. Take about 7–10 frozen cubes and some fresh juice and blend together to make a delicious fruit slush or another healthful dessert. I also put the frozen cubes through my Champion Juicer for the perfect sorbet.

FAT-FREE ITALIAN RASPBERRY DRESSING

No oil is needed because the vegetables emulsify the dressing.
Makes about 2½ cups.

1 small red onion, peeled, cored and cut into quarters
1 medium red pepper, seeded and cut into quarters
1 large yellow pepper, seeded and cut into quarters
½ cup raspberry vinegar
½ cup water or more, as needed
⅓ cup brown-rice syrup or agave nectar
1 Tbsp. finely chopped fresh oregano
2 tsp. minced garlic

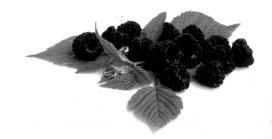

1 tsp. finely chopped fresh chervil
1 tsp. finely chopped fresh tarragon
1 tsp. fresh lemon juice
Dash of salt

Blend all ingredients in a blender or food processor at high speed for 1 minute. Keep in the refrigerator. Use within 2 days. Mix well before using.

SWEET PEPPER–APPLE DRESSING

This recipe is wonderful for your skin (and waistline).
Makes about 2 cups.

1 cup fresh apple juice
½ cup chopped apple
½ cup chopped sweet bell pepper (red, yellow, or orange)
½ cup sunflower seeds, soaked for 8 hours or overnight in enough water to
     amply cover the seeds
1 Tbsp. flaxseeds, soaked for 8 hours or overnight in enough water to amply
     cover the seeds
1½ tsp. dried dill

Drain the seeds. Blend all ingredients in a blender or food processor until smooth. Serve immediately. Keep in the refrigerator. Use within 2–3 days, and be sure to mix before using.

GREEN-GODDESS DRESSING

Here's another marvelous topping for potatoes, steamed vegetables, or grain dishes and dip for vegetables, in addition to dressing crisp green salads. It's guaranteed to bring out the goddess in you to get your family to worship and appreciate you!
Makes about 2 cups.

1 large ripe avocado, peeled, pitted, and cut into quarters
1 small red onion, peeled, cored, and cut into quarters
2 celery stalks, juiced
1 cucumber, peeled and cut into quarters
¼ cup fresh parsley
¼ cup fresh dill
¼ cup fresh basil
¼ cup watercress
1 small clove garlic, minced
1–2 tsp. fresh lemon juice
½ tsp. lemon zest (from an organic lemon only)
Low-sodium tamari or sea salt to taste

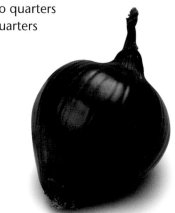

Blend all ingredients in a blender or food processor until smooth. Use extra celery juice to reach desired consistency. Keep in the refrigerator. Use within 2 days.

LEMONY RANCH DRESSING

Here's a healthier version than most store-bought ranch dressings that doubles as a vegetable dip or topping on potatoes.
Makes almost 2 cups.

8 oz. firm lite organic silken tofu, cubed (or 8 oz. plain nondairy yogurt)
¼ cup Lemonaise Spread (see Chapter 4)
¼ cup purified water
3 scallions, finely chopped
2 Tbsp. fresh lemon juice
1–2 cloves garlic, minced
1 Tbsp. chopped fresh parsley
2 tsp. chopped fresh dill
1 tsp. chopped fresh oregano
1 tsp. ground cumin
1 tsp. sea salt

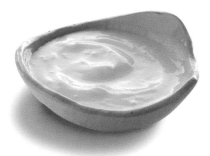

Blend all ingredients in a blender or food processor until smooth. Keep in the refrigerator. Use within 4–5 days.

PEAR-CASHEW-CREAM DRESSING

This is a superb dressing for fruit and other desserts. It also makes a delicious dip for strawberries and apple quarters.

Makes about 3 cups.

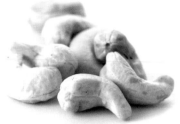

2 pears
2 cups water
1 cup raw cashews
⅛ tsp. cinnamon

Peel and dice pears. Blend all ingredients in a blender or food processor until smooth. Chill. Use within 4–5 days.

GRAPEFRUIT-MUSTARD DRESSING

One of my favorite fruits, grapefruit gives this dressing a flavorful punch.
Makes about ⅓ cup.

1 Tbsp. Bragg Liquid Aminos
1 Tbsp. fresh grapefruit juice
2 tsp. fresh lemon juice
1½ Tbsp. flaxseed oil or cold-pressed, extra-virgin olive oil
1–2 cloves garlic, pressed
1 tsp. Dijon mustard

Combine all ingredients in a bowl and whisk well. Use within 2 days.

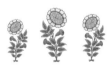

CHAPTER 7

SOUPS

"Eat to live, don't live to eat . . . many dishes, many diseases."

— BENJAMIN FRANKLIN

Whether hot or cold or as an appetizer, snack, or main meal, soups can be a great way to provide a nutrient-rich, satisfying dish without too many calories. Like a green salad, if you have a cup or bowl of soup before your main course, it will help fill you up so that you don't overeat. And as the main course, soup can be a delicious entrée that won't leave you with that stuffed feeling.

Soups are a much better on-the-go meal than anything from a fast-food restaurant. Just fill up a thermos and take some soup with you when you leave for work, run errands, go to school, or head to the beach. You can make legume, fruit, or vegetable varieties and even dessert soups—the sky's the limit! Most freeze beautifully, so they're a practical way to always have something healthful and delicious on hand.

Experimenting with Soups

In addition to varying the ingredients of the recipes to create new favorites, you can experiment with different serving temperatures. When the weather outside is frosty, I like to dunk whole-grain breads or chips into my hot soup to make the meal more filling (see Chapter 16). When the weather is warm, I like to eat my soups chilled, accompanied by raw vegetables and a light dip (see Chapter 4).

Enjoy these healthful soup recipes. And remember, the possibilities for creativity are endless!

VEGETABLE BROTH

This quick, easy, versatile base can be used in so many ways: by itself or as the liquid for grains, dressings, dips, and sauces. Any recipe that calls for chicken broth can be made successfully with vegetable broth. When you cut the vegetables into small pieces, about ½ inch or smaller, their flavor will saturate the liquid in only 20 minutes. I usually triple the recipe and freeze it in one-cup containers or in freezer-quality zip-top bags so that I always have it on hand. By making your own, you can ensure that only the highest-quality organic vegetables are used, and you'll also keep the sodium level down.

Makes 8 cups.

8 cups purified water
1 red onion
1 yellow onion
3 carrots, peeled and diced
4 stalks celery, diced
2 cups sliced shiitake mushrooms
2 parsnips, peeled and diced
1 turnip, peeled and diced
1 leek, white and pale green parts only, diced
3 large cloves garlic, minced
1 strip of kombu, approximately 4 inches in length
1 bay leaf
6 sprigs parsley
3 whole cloves
1 tsp. whole coriander seed

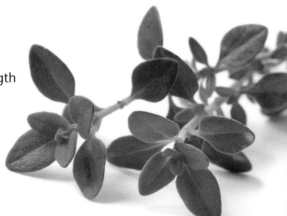

In a large pot, combine all ingredients, bring to a boil (remove the kombu just before the water boils), lower heat, and simmer for 20 minutes, uncovered. Strain through a fine sieve or a double thickness of cheesecloth.

Variation: Create a bouquet garni with the fresh herbs by filling a celery or fennel stalk with sprigs of fresh herbs such as thyme, oregano, tarragon, rosemary, basil, chervil, or parsley, and tying it with a cotton thread or string. Leave a long tail so you can remove it easily before serving.

FYI: Thyme

Thyme's aromatic oil contains two chemicals: thymol and carvacrol. Both have preservative, antibacterial, and antifungal properties. They can also act as expectorants (phlegm loosening) and may be useful as digestive aids. As an antiseptic, thyme fights several disease-causing bacteria and fungi. Pregnant women may use thyme as a culinary spice, but they should avoid large amounts and shouldn't use the herb's oil.

POTASSIUM-POWERED BROTH

This delicious alkaline broth is a natural diuretic that I use as a soup base or beverage, and I often include the liquid when cooking grains or casseroles.

Makes 12–14 cups.

10 cups purified water
2½ lbs. russet, red, and Yukon Gold potatoes, washed and cut into
    ½-inch chunks
2 cups chopped green cabbage
1½ cups chopped broccoli, stalks and florets
5 large carrots, diced
2 red onions, diced
1 yellow onion, diced
1 bunch celery (including leaves), chopped
2 cloves garlic, minced
Fresh bouquet garni (see preceding Vegetable Broth recipe)

In a large pot, combine all ingredients and bring to a boil. Reduce heat and simmer for 1½ hours, uncovered. Strain through a fine sieve. You can keep it in your refrigerator for 3–5 days, or freeze in 1–2 cup containers for future use.

SHIITAKE CONSOMMÉ WITH GREENS

This simple, rejuvenating, immune-boosting soup is always a winner, especially if you're under extra stress or need an energy enhancer.

Serves 4–6.

7 cups Vegetable Broth (see recipe earlier in this chapter)
1 cup thinly sliced fresh shiitake mushrooms (or ⅔ cup dried)
1 Tbsp. unrefined sesame oil (optional)
2 cloves garlic, minced
1 lb. chopped greens (such as chard, kale, collard, or mustard)
1 Tbsp. white miso
2 tsp. lemon juice
1 tsp. lime juice

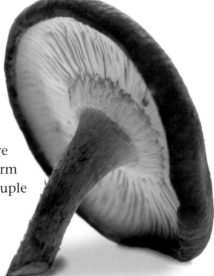

In a large stockpot, heat the Vegetable Broth. While the broth is heating, sauté the garlic and mushrooms with the oil in a skillet until slightly tender, 3–4 minutes. Add sauté mixture to the stockpot. Then add the greens and simmer for about 12–15 minutes. Place ½ cup of the soup stock in a small bowl. Dissolve the lime and lemon juices and miso into this warm stock. Mix back into the soup and heat for a couple of minutes, but don't boil. Serve hot.

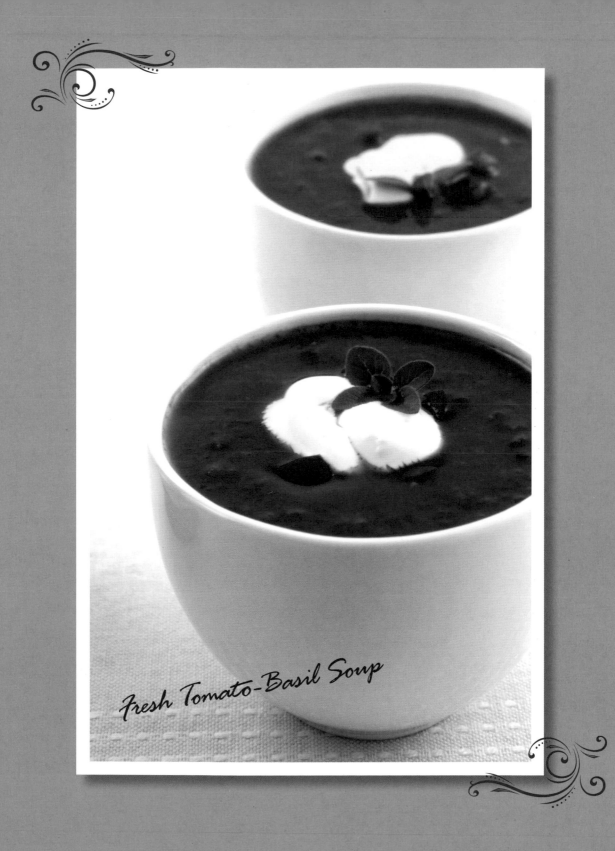

Fresh Tomato-Basil Soup

Tip: Shiitake Mushrooms

The shiitake mushrooms have long been used in Chinese and Japanese cooking and are known for their medicinal properties of strengthening the immune system and restoring youthful vitality. Their chewy, firm texture and woodsy taste make them particularly satisfying in meatless cooking. I add them to soups, vegetable stews, stir-fries, veggie burgers, and pasta sauces. When buying fresh, look for firm ones with a nice aroma and refrigerate them in a single layer on a small tray, covered with a dampened towel so that they'll keep for a few days. Dried shiitake must be softened first in water: hot water for half an hour, or cold for several hours. Make sure to use the flavorful soaking liquid, too.

FRESH TOMATO-BASIL SOUP

This easy-to-prepare soup freezes well and is good hot or cold. Make it in the summer, when tomato season is at its height.

Serves 3–6.

4 lbs. fresh ripe tomatoes, peeled, seeded, and coarsely chopped
½ cup Vegetable Broth (see recipe earlier in this chapter)
¼ cup diced onion
1 clove garlic, pressed
Sea salt to taste
⅓ cup finely chopped fresh basil, for garnish

In a medium nonreactive saucepan, combine tomatoes, broth, onion, garlic, and salt to taste. Bring to a boil, reduce heat to medium-low, and cook just until the onions are tender, about 12–15 minutes. Serve garnished with the chopped basil.

Variations: If you have time, lightly sauté the onion and garlic in 1 Tbsp. extra-virgin olive oil; add to the soup 5 minutes before it's finished. You can use other freshly chopped herbs such as cilantro, oregano, Italian parsley, chives, or mint. If you like garlic, try adding 2–3 large cloves, minced. To increase protein and enhance the basil flavor, blend 3 oz. lite organic silken tofu with 3 Tbsp. Vegetable Broth and ¼ cup extra basil. Add this mixture to the soup during the last 5 minutes of cooking so that it's heated throughout. Top with homemade croutons (see Chapter 16) and a dollop of plain nondairy yogurt.

SWEET SQUASH & PARSNIP SOUP

You'll become an instant lover of squash and parsnips with this great-tasting, easy-to-prepare soup.

Serves 2–4.

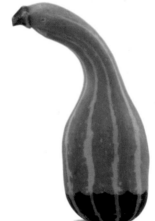

5 crookneck squash, chopped
4 medium zucchini, chopped
6 parsnips, chopped
⅓–½ cup purified water, Vegetable Broth
    (see recipe earlier in this chapter), or nut milk
⅓ cup fresh parsley, chopped
¼ cup fresh orange juice
1 Tbsp. rice syrup
½ tsp. Bragg Liquid Aminos
Dash ground cardamom

In separate pans, steam the squash and parsnips until tender (they take different lengths of time to steam). In a blender or food processor, purée the squash and parsnips with the other ingredients and enough liquid to create the desired consistency. Reheat and garnish with fresh parsley.

Variations: Substitute cinnamon for cardamom. For added protein and a creamier soup, blend in 3 oz. organic silken tofu with some of the liquid and stir into the soup, heating through. If you don't eat soy products, blend together ¼ cup cashews with some of the liquid and stir into the soup. To make it richer, blend ½ avocado with some liquid and stir it into the soup.

SIMPLE FRESH CORN & AVOCADO SOUP

This light, uncooked soup would make a perfect snack or side dish for a summer evening.
Serves 2.

1 cup vegetable juice (mixture of carrot, celery, romaine lettuce, and 1–2 green onions)
1 large ear of fresh corn, cut off the cob
1 small avocado
Sea salt to taste
Freshly chopped cilantro, parsley, or chives as garnish

Blend all ingredients in a blender or food processor. Serve chilled, at room temperature, or warmed. Garnish with fresh herbs.
Variation: I'll sometimes blend only half of the soup, so it remains a little crunchy. Also, try adding chopped green onions or other favorite chopped vegetables to the blended soup in order to enhance the texture.

FYI: Corn

Corn offers so many nutrients, including iron, zinc, and potassium, not to mention lots of fiber. We think of corn as a vegetable, but it's really a grain. Mixed with legumes, it provides a complete protein. When cooking the kernels, never add salt to the water because it toughens them. My favorite way to eat corn is freshly picked, right off the cob or with the raw kernels cut into my salad for added color, flavor, and crunchiness (plus extra nutrients). Plus, this wonderful food has only 75 calories per ear or ½ cup (raw), or 90 calories (cooked).

PAPAYA GAZPACHO

Everything about this chilled soup—the color, the taste, and the easy preparation—makes this unique dish a wonderful appetizer, snack, or meal.
Caution: Habanero chilis are among the hottest peppers you can eat, so always wear latex gloves when handling them.
Serves 3–6.

2 cups (2 lbs.) ripe papaya, cut into chunks and chilled

⅔ cup freshly squeezed orange juice

½–1 tsp. fresh habanero chili (or 1–2 tsp. fresh red Fresno chili), seeded and minced

⅔ cup Vegetable Broth (see recipe earlier in this chapter)

⅓ cup fresh lime juice

2 tsp. fresh lemon juice

⅓ cup chopped green onions

¾ cup ripe (but still firm) avocado, peeled and diced into ¼-inch pieces

3 Tbsp. chopped fresh cilantro or parsley, for garnish

Sea salt to taste

First, set aside about ½ cup of the papaya and cut into ½-inch dice for garnish. In a blender or food processor, combine the remaining papaya chunks, orange juice, and chili, and blend until smooth. Transfer this mixture into a bowl. Add the Vegetable Broth, lime and lemon juices, and green onions, and stir to combine. Add salt to taste. Chill in the refrigerator for 4–8 hours. To serve, pour or ladle the liquid into individual serving bowls. In each bowl, add equal portions of the green onions, ripe papaya, and avocado. Sprinkle with fresh herbs and adjust salt to taste.

MEAL-IN-A-BOWL WHITE-BEAN SOUP

This hearty soup is both filling and delicious.
Serves 3–6.

1 cup uncooked dry navy beans

2 tsp. cold-pressed, extra-virgin olive oil

1 large red onion, diced

3 large cloves garlic, minced

3–4 large Yukon Gold (or your favorite) potatoes, cut into ½-inch dice

3 medium carrots, cut into ¼-inch slices

2 medium stalks celery, cut into ¼-inch slices

¾ cup shredded red cabbage

¾ cup shredded green cabbage

3 cups Vegetable Broth (see recipe earlier in this chapter)

3 cups purified water

1 large bay leaf

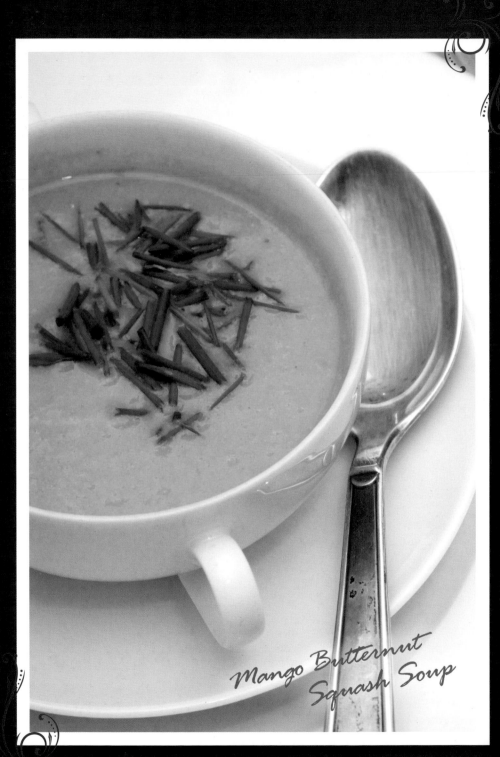

Mango Butternut
Squash Soup

In a medium bowl, cover the beans with enough water to submerge them by 2 inches and soak for 2 hours. Drain and rinse, discarding the soaking water. In a large stockpot, heat oil over medium heat. Add the onion and sauté until tender, about 5–7 minutes. Add garlic and sauté for another minute or two, stirring constantly. Add the remaining ingredients and bring to a boil. Reduce heat to low and simmer for about 60–70 minutes, or until the beans are tender. Add more water to create the desired consistency.

Variation: For added minerals and flavor, add a 4-inch strip of kombu when simmering. Remove before serving.

FYI: Legumes

Legumes, aka beans, are very low in fat and brimming with soluble fiber that helps lower cholesterol and normalize blood-sugar levels. They're an excellent source of protein and iron and are rich in vitamins and minerals such as potassium and calcium. If consumed regularly, beans can lower cholesterol and are a good source of plant protein.

MANGO-BUTTERNUT-SQUASH SOUP

The delightful combination of mangos and butternut squash gives this soup an especially rich and beautiful color and packs it with vitamin A.

Serves 3–5.

3 cups butternut squash, peeled, seeded, and chopped (lightly steamed
    until just tender)
1 large ripe mango, seeded and cubed
3¼ cups fresh orange juice
¾ cup fresh apple juice
⅓ cup (about 3–4) pitted dates
1 Tbsp. fresh lime juice
2 tsp. curry powder
1 tsp. lemon zest (from an organic lemon only)
Sprigs of mint, diced mango, or other garnish

Blend all ingredients in a blender or food processor until creamy smooth. Garnish and serve hot, warm, or chilled.

FYI: Mangos

One of my favorite tropical fruits, juicy mangos are perhaps best eaten in the shower—either alone or with someone special—because they can be quite messy. They contain more than a full day's supply of vitamin A in the form of beta-carotene, as well as lots of vitamin C. Their fat content is barely detectable, and there are only 130 calories per 7-oz. serving. The versatile mango makes a great snack and a delicious breakfast when combined with papaya and kiwi; it can also be added to smoothies.

POTATO-LEEK SOUP

Hot or chilled, here's a delicious way to add health-promoting leeks to your diet. You can easily double the batch and freeze the extra in 1½-cup containers.

Serves 2–4.

2 tsp. cold-pressed, extra-virgin olive oil
4 large leek stalks, sliced
1 medium red onion, diced
1 clove garlic, minced
2 cups water
2 cups Vegetable Broth (see recipe earlier in this chapter)
4 large Yukon Gold (or your favorite) potatoes, diced
1½ tsp. low-sodium tamari
¼ cup fresh tarragon, minced

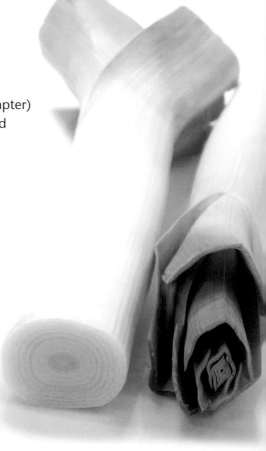

In a large stockpot, heat the oil and sauté garlic, onion, and leeks over medium heat for about 6–7 minutes. Add the broth, water, potatoes, and tamari. Simmer for about 15 minutes or until the potatoes and leeks are soft. Transfer ¾ cup of the mixture to a blender or food processor and blend until smooth. Return to the pot. Add the tarragon and stir well. Serve as is, or purée with a hand blender for a creamy, smooth texture. Serve hot, warm, or chilled.

HOT-N-SPICY MISO-TOFU SOUP

This Asian-style dish uses the traditional soy in three ways: miso, tofu, and tamari. It's a little saltier than most of my soups (due to the miso and tamari), but it packs a real protein punch. If you don't eat soy products or choose to limit them in your diet, as I do, please refer to my book *Be Healthy~Stay Balanced* for recipes to make nondairy yogurt, milk, and cheese; and tofu-like products from nuts, seeds, and grains.

Serves 4–6.

½ cup Vegetable Broth (see recipe earlier in this chapter)
1 large onion, thinly sliced
4 slices ginger (¼-inch thick)
2 cloves garlic, minced
8 cups water
½ lb. firm organic tofu (⅔ cup), cubed
2 Tbsp. low-sodium tamari
2 Tbsp. rice vinegar
3 medium carrots, sliced diagonally
1 strip of kombu (about 6 inches)
3 Tbsp. red miso
1–2 tsp. freshly ground black pepper
Dash cayenne

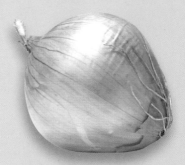

In a large stockpot, steam-sauté the onions, garlic, and ginger in the Vegetable Broth, until the onions are translucent. Add the water, tofu, carrots, kombu, tamari, and vinegar. Gently simmer until the kombu is soft, about 15–20 minutes. Take out the kombu, cut it into thick strips, and return them to the pot. Right before serving, scoop out one cup of the broth, dissolve the miso in the broth, then return to the pot for a minute (do not boil). Add the pepper and the cayenne and stir well. Serve hot.

FYI: Miso

Fresh miso is a fermented paste made from soybeans and other legumes and grains that can be used as a stock base for risotto, soups, and sauces. Because miso is partially digested by fermentation, the body easily assimilates its nutrients. Miso also contains live enzymes that benefit the microbial balance of the digestive tract. It provides anticancer properties without any of the chemicals often found in stock cubes and powders. The lighter color misos, such as white or yellow, are more mellow in flavor than the darker ones.

ZESTY ROASTED-YELLOW-PEPPER & ORANGE SOUP

Whether for a family picnic or a romantic dinner for two, this colorful soup is always a winner.

Serves 2–4.

3 yellow roasted bell peppers, chopped (see Chapter 16)
1 yellow onion, chopped
½ cup fresh orange juice
1¾ cups Vegetable Broth (see recipe earlier in this chapter)
Grated rind of one organic orange
1 jalapeno pepper, seeds and white ribs removed, minced
Dash of nutmeg
Sea salt to taste
Freshly chopped parsley or chives for garnish

In a medium pan, sauté the onion in 2 Tbsp. of the orange juice until onions are tender, about 5 minutes, stirring often. In a blender or food processor, combine the roasted peppers, sautéed onion, remaining orange juice, half the orange rind, the vegetable broth, and jalapeno pepper. Blend until smooth. Add the nutmeg; season to taste with salt. Heat until warm throughout, about 2–3 minutes. Garnish with the fresh herbs and serve right away.

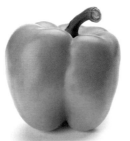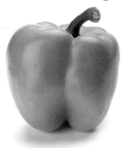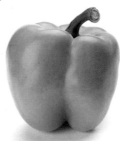

SAVORY GINGER-WINTER-SQUASH SOUP

Ginger gives this winter soup its extra zip and wonderful warming properties. Serves 3–4.

1 large winter squash, peeled, seeded, and cut into 1-inch pieces
1 cup plain almond milk (see Chapter 2)
1¼-inch piece fresh ginger, peeled and juiced
½ tsp. sea salt
2 cups Vegetable Broth (see recipe earlier in this chapter)
3 Tbsp. minced fresh chives

In a large pot, combine the squash, milk, Vegetable Broth, and ginger. Bring to a boil. Reduce heat and simmer until squash is tender. Add salt to taste and mix well. Let soup cool slightly, then transfer to a blender or food processor and purée until smooth. Pour into individual soup bowls and garnish with fresh chives. This is equally good warm or chilled.

FYI: Squash

Squash is a wonderful low-calorie and highly nutritious food. Rich in calcium, magnesium, potassium, beta-carotene, and vitamin C, squash helps relieve acidosis because of its alkalinity. It's also rich in alpha lipoic acid, a powerful antioxidant that helps prevent wrinkles and reverse the aging process. I even put raw squash in my smoothies.

BLACK-BEAN STEW/SOUP

With its lemongrass and cilantro accents, this black-bean soup has a distinctly Southeast Asian flavor.
Serves 6–8.

2 cups dry black beans or 6 cups cooked black beans
1 large onion, chopped
1 cup chopped carrots (2–3 carrots)
1 cup chopped celery (2–3 stalks)
2–3 large cloves garlic, pressed

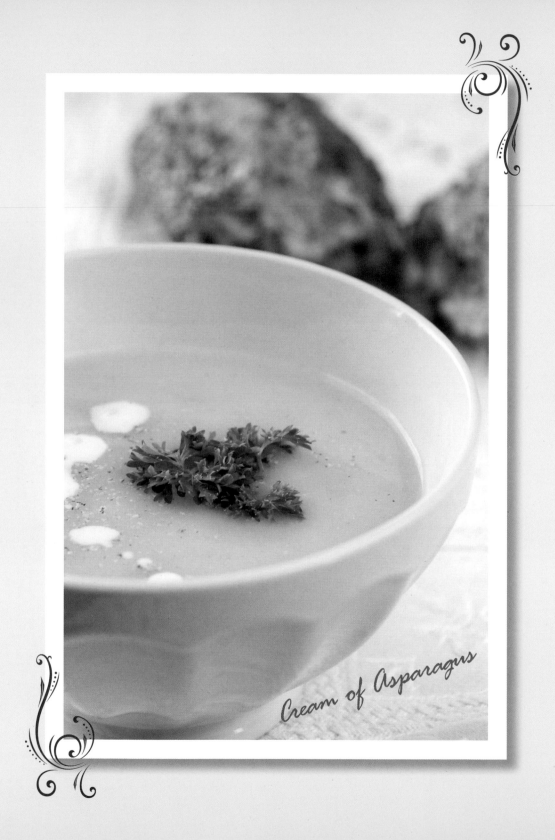

Cream of Asparagus

1 tsp. cold-pressed, extra-virgin olive oil
4 cups Vegetable Broth (see recipe earlier in this chapter)
3 Tbsp. fresh cilantro, chopped
1 Tbsp. fresh thyme, chopped
1 tsp. sea salt
Dash cayenne pepper

If using dry beans, soak 2 cups overnight; then drain, rinse, cover with water, and cook until tender. If using canned beans, drain and rinse 6 cups and set aside. In a large stockpot, sauté onion, carrots, celery, and garlic in the olive oil and 1 Tbsp. Vegetable Broth. Add 1 cup broth along with the cooked beans and combine everything thoroughly. Simmer 10 minutes, covered, stirring occasionally. Add the herbs, salt, and dash of cayenne pepper, and simmer 10 more minutes. You can stop here, as this makes a delicious black-bean stew. For a soup consistency, add the rest of the broth and simmer 10 minutes more.

Variations: For a creamy soup, blend 6 oz. organic silken tofu with 3 ladles (about 2 cups) of the soup mixture (liquid, beans, and veggies) until smooth. Return mixture to the stockpot and simmer a few more minutes. For an even creamier version, blend the entire soup mixture with 9 oz. tofu. Return to the stockpot and simmer a few minutes more. In my book *Be Healthy~Stay Balanced,* I offer many additional recipes for substitutes for soy products.

CREAM OF ASPARAGUS

Asparagus fans rejoice: this fabulous soup takes fewer than 30 minutes to make!
Serves 4–6.

4 cups Vegetable Broth (see recipe earlier in this chapter)
2 cups chopped fresh asparagus
⅓ cup chopped Maui or other sweet onion
1 cup plain nondairy yogurt
Sea salt to taste
Freshly chopped cilantro, parsley, or chives, for garnish

In a medium saucepan, heat the broth. Add the onion and asparagus and cook over medium heat until soft, about 10 minutes. Cool slightly. In a food processor or blender, purée the soup in 3–4 batches. Return to the saucepan, add the nondairy yogurt, and gently reheat. Salt to taste and garnish with fresh herbs. Serve immediately.

Variations: Substitute broccoli, carrots, brussels sprouts, or cauliflower for the asparagus.

FYI: Asparagus

Four spears of asparagus have only 13 calories! Asparagus is chock-full of iron, protein, potassium, calcium, magnesium, selenium, beta-carotene, and vitamins A and K. One of nature's most complete vegetables, this gourmet delight also contains asparagine, which stimulates the kidneys. Asparagine gives the spears their diuretic qualities and also gives certain people's urine a characteristic odor just minutes after eating. (These folks lack the gene needed to break asparagine down, but there's no harm in that, as I know personally.) Studies at the University of California and the Mount Sinai School of Medicine in New York have linked regular asparagus consumption to dramatically lower rates of cancer and heart disease. According to the National Cancer Institute, it's the food highest in glutathione, an important anticarcinogen. *Caution:* Asparagus contains purine, so avoid it if you suffer from gout.

FYI: Glutathione

Glutathione is your body's master antioxidant and has the ability to neutralize free-radical damage. For more information on my favorite glutathione-accelerating nutritional supplement that I wouldn't be without, see Chapter 11.

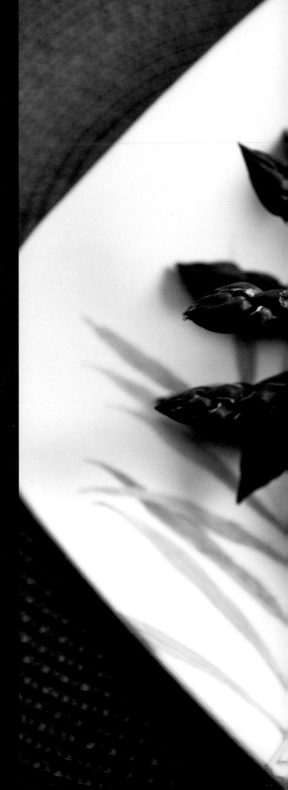

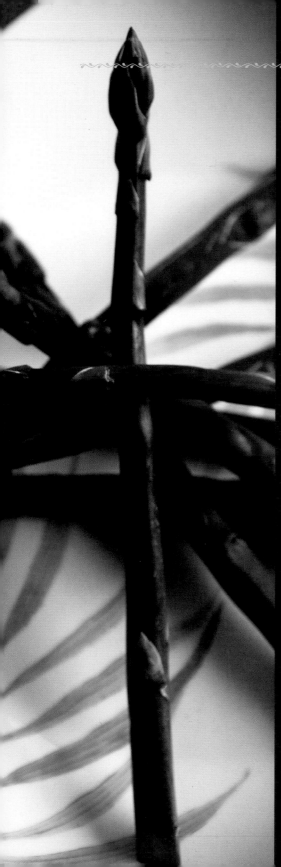

CHILLED CANTALOUPE-LIME SOUP

This raw and refreshing soup is perfect on a hot summer day!

Serves 3–6.

2 ripe cantaloupes, cut into chunks
1 cup fresh orange juice (or tangerine or combination)
⅓ cup fresh lime juice
1 tsp. grated fresh ginger root
½ organic lime, thinly sliced
4–6 fresh mint sprigs

In a food processor or blender, purée the melon, orange juice, lime juice, and ginger. Pour into serving bowls and chill in the bowls. Garnish each serving with a slice of lime and a sprig of mint.

Variations: Substitute honeydew or crenshaw melon for the cantaloupe and fresh apple, peach, nectarine, or strawberry juice for the orange juice.

FYI: Melons

Melons have one of the highest fiber contents of any food. Add to this large amounts of vitamins A and C, plus more than 800 milligrams of potassium in half a cantaloupe. One day a week, try eating just melon for a great and easy cleanse and rejuvenator. When buying cantaloupe, look for fine, even netting, even if the melon requires a few days to ripen. The finer the netting, the sweeter the flesh. With only 50 calories per cup, melon is your friend.

CURRIED SPLIT-PEA SOUP

This quickly will become your favorite split-pea soup.
Serves 6–10.

6 cups Vegetable Broth (see recipe earlier in
    this chapter)
6 cups purified water
1 lb. organic split peas
3 medium carrots, diced
3 stalks celery, diced
1 large Maui or sweet red onion, diced
2 cloves garlic, minced
2 large bay leaves
2 tsp. curry powder
2 tsp. sea salt (optional)

Rinse peas well in a strainer, and make sure
to discard any stones. In a large stockpot, bring
the broth and water to a boil. Add the peas,
return to a boil, reduce heat, and cover. Simmer, stirring occasionally, for about 30 minutes. Skim off any foam
that accumulates on the top. Add onion, celery, carrots, garlic, bay
leaves, curry powder, and salt. Continue to simmer for 45–50 minutes, stirring
occasionally. Adjust seasonings to taste and serve.

Variation: Substitute yellow split peas or lentils for the green split peas.

CAULIFLOWER-CARROT SOUP WITH TARRAGON

Simply delicious, and oh so good for you.
Serves 4–6.

3 cups Vegetable Broth (see recipe earlier in this chapter)
1 large onion, finely diced
1–2 cloves garlic, finely minced
2¼ cups (1½ lbs.) carrots, peeled and cut into ½-inch dice

1⅓ cups (¾ lb.) Yukon Gold (or russet) potatoes,
    peeled and cut into ½-inch dice
2 green onions, finely chopped
1¼ cups purified water
2 cups (1 lb.) cauliflower, in small florets
⅓ cup (2 oz.) lite organic silken tofu or alternative non-soy product
1 Tbsp. chopped fresh tarragon

In a stockpot, combine ¼ cup Vegetable Broth, onion, and garlic. Cover and simmer over medium heat until onion is translucent, about 5–7 minutes. Add the carrots, potatoes, green onions, remaining Vegetable Broth, and water. Bring to a boil. Lower the heat and simmer for about 5 minutes. Add the cauliflower, cover and simmer for about 15 more minutes, or until all vegetables are tender. Cool slightly, then transfer to a blender and purée with the tofu. Return to stockpot and add tarragon. Stir about 1–2 more minutes over low heat. If desired, add more water. Season to taste and serve.

Variation: Substitute broccoflower, a pale green cauliflower-broccoli hybrid, for the cauliflower to create a lovely color and delicious soup.

FYI: Cauliflower

This extremely low-calorie member of the cabbage family has virtually no fat or sodium, so you can eat as much of it as you want. A one-cup serving provides 100 percent of the RDA for vitamin C, and it's also rich in phosphorus. The National Academy of Sciences singled out cauliflower as one of the best cancer-prevention foods.

FYI: Tarragon

Like many culinary herbs, the oil in tarragon fights disease-causing bacteria. For garden first aid, press some freshly crushed tarragon leaves onto wounds on your way to washing and bandaging them. The oil contains an anesthetic chemical, eugenol, which is the major constituent of anesthetic clove oil, supporting its age-old use for toothache.

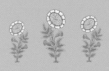

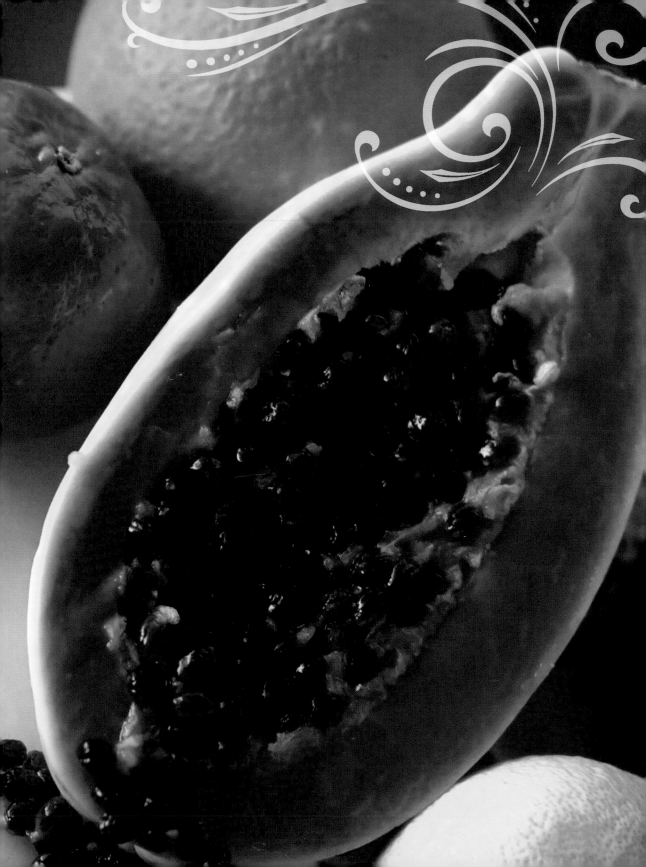

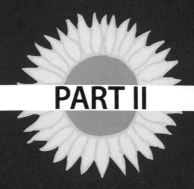

PART II

LIVING
VIBRANT

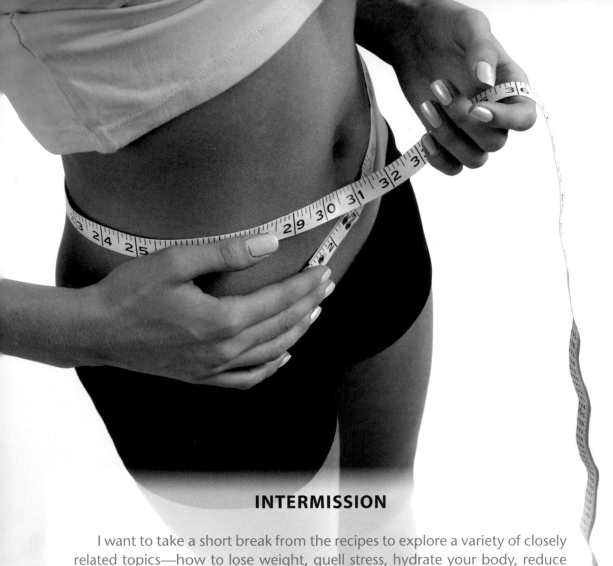

INTERMISSION

I want to take a short break from the recipes to explore a variety of closely related topics—how to lose weight, quell stress, hydrate your body, reduce inflammation, and heal with sprouts. I've also included a special chapter on raising healthy children.

CHAPTER 8

WEIGHT LOSS MADE EASY:
REACHING & MAINTAINING YOUR IDEAL WEIGHT

"Regardless of our body size, self-respect and self-acceptance are the starting points for making peace with our size. We must know that we have the power to get off the weight treadmill and start enjoying our life, no matter where we are."

— Christiane Northrup, M.D.

While millions are starving to death around the world, Americans have the dubious honor of being the fattest people on the globe. Is it any wonder that we're preoccupied with our waistlines? U.S. residents spend more than $40 billion a year on diet foods, programs, pills, and other "guaranteed" weight-loss regimens and products. Yet according to the National Center for Health Statistics, we're getting fatter all the time.

Experts call obesity an American epidemic—one that brings with it major health problems. Heart disease, endometrial (uterine) and breast cancer, high cholesterol, high blood pressure, immune dysfunction, osteoarthritis, stroke, gout, sleep disorders, gallstones, and diabetes are all associated with obesity. Since I'm always looking at the glass half full and choose to discern things from an optimistic point of view (that's why I got my nickname "Sunny"), let's put this in a more positive way: *losing even a little weight will improve your health and well-being significantly—and help prevent those very same diseases.*

Undereating is also a problem, and disorders such as anorexia and bulimia are on the rise. Advertising for women's clothing contributes to the problem by using models who look like waifs. Consider Barbie, a doll that's part of most little girls' upbringing. This model of good looks and the "perfect body" is giving the wrong message about what a healthy woman should look like. Were Barbie an actual person, her body fat would be so low that she probably wouldn't even menstruate. As girls treasure the doll and teens try to emulate her, she has one accessory that's consistently missing—food.

Surveys indicate that most people are unhappy with their weight or the shape of their bodies. Currently, half of the women and a quarter of the men in the United States are trying to lose weight and reshape themselves. The sad thing is that the majority are going about it in the wrong way, the hard way—by dieting, which doesn't work! Throw away books that say you can eat whatever you want and still lose weight and keep it off, or that you can expect long-lasting success without exercising. Dieting isn't the cure. After you finish such a program, you may have lost some fat, but *you haven't lost the tendency to get fat.*

Obesity, Diabetes & Insalubrity

Obesity and type 2 diabetes are near epidemic levels, as nearly two-thirds of the adult population is overweight. The 2003–2004 National Health and Nutrition Examination Survey (NHANES) data on the prevalence of overweight and obesity among adults reveals to us that noninstitutionalized adults age 20 years and over who are overweight and/or obese make up 66.3 percent of the U.S. population. The percentage of adults age 20 years and over who are obese is 32 percent.

Seventeen percent of adolescents ages 12 to 19 are overweight, as are 19 percent of children ages 6 to 11. In his book *Eat to Live,* Joel Furhman, M.D., states: "The number one health problem in the United States is obesity, and if the current trend continues, by the year 2030 all adults in the United States will be obese."

A study in the July 2008 issue of *American Journal of Epidemiology* (2008; 168:30–37) found that people who were obese or overweight in adolescence were three to four times as likely to have died of heart disease by middle age as compared with their thinner peers.

What does the future hold in terms of health and quality of life if this epidemic isn't halted? Is there a way for individuals struggling with weight issues to take control of their health and permanently shed those unwanted, life-threatening pounds? The answer is a resounding *yes!* In these pages, we'll look at some of the causes and the consequences of the current obesity epidemic, and how each individual who chooses to do so can take control and win the battle of the bulge and declining health. So please stay with me; you'll be glad you did.

A recent article in *USA Today* (January 24, 2008) stated:

> Uncontrolled diabetes wreaks havoc on the body, often leading to kidney failure, blindness, and death. A new study shows that the nation's unchecked diabetes epidemic exacts a heavy financial toll as well: $174 billion a year. That is about as much as the conflicts in Iraq, Afghanistan, and the global war on terrorism combined. It is more than the $150 billion in damages caused by Hurricane Katrina.
>
> The incidence of diabetes has ballooned—there are one million new cases a year—as more Americans become overweight or obese. The cost of diabetes—both in direct medical care and lost productivity—has swelled 32 percent since 2002. And, diabetes killed more than 284,000 Americans last year.

What Causes This Weighty Issue?

Over the last few decades, the population in general has moved further and further away from a diet rich in plant-based foods to one centered around commercially produced animal products and low- to no-fiber sugar-enhanced processed foods, refined grains, and fast foods that provide little nutritional value and an excess of calories. Not only do these caloric-rich, nutrient-poor foods contribute to excess weight, but they also contribute to insulin resistance and other hormone-related issues.

Americans as well as most of the industrialized world have a love affair with rich foods that are nutrient-deficient and disease-causing. Even in biblical days, people were instructed regarding the consumption of a diet that was filled with rich foods. Proverbs 23:1–3 says: "When you sit to dine with a ruler, note well what is before you, and put a knife to your throat if you are given to gluttony. Do not crave his delicacies, for that food is deceptive." Wow. There's no mincing of words there. And in the days of Solomon, the principle author of Proverbs, only rulers could afford the luxuries of rich foods. The common person could partake of them only on special occasions.

I find it remarkable that even thousands of years ago, there was a warning to be careful with rich foods because they're "deceptive." They satisfy the taste buds, become addictive, and don't support optimal health. Most Americans today eat like kings three times each day or more, 365 days of the year, and are reaping the consequences of their poor choices.

In *Inflammation Nation,* Floyd H. Chilton, Ph.D., discusses the obesity connection to inflammation and other diseases. He states:

> Inflammatory disease and obesity are not simply maladies running on parallel tracks, but are intrinsically intertwined for a number of reasons. There are a number of straightforward connections between those excess pounds and inflammatory disease.
>
> One of those commonalities is what I call "foods of affluence" and the overwhelming quantities of some of those foods in the typical Western diet. For instance, early humans obtained more than half of their calories from carbohydrates, but most of these carbohydrates came from vegetables and fruit, with a smattering of beans and whole grains thrown in. In affluent societies, carbohydrates take the form of refined, added sugars and highly processed grain flours, highly caloric foods that provide us none of the nutrients necessary for optimal health. The ready availability of eggs, meat, and poultry is another function of our affluence.

When we look around us, almost all social events are centered around food—dishes that have little if any nutritional value, but that appeal to the taste buds. If we're ever to overcome the epidemic of overweight and obesity, we must change the way we look at food. We should be making wise choices that support optimal health, eating to live and not living to eat.

Maybe It's Not All in Your Genes

Children whose parents are obese have a tenfold increased risk of being obese as well. While the parents' condition sets a predisposition for their kids, it's the combination of food choices, inactivity, and genetic tendencies that determine obesity. Can we blame genetics for the problem? On June 16, 2008, Reuters News published an article titled "Healthy Lifestyle Triggers Genetic Changes," which described a three-month, groundbreaking study led by Dean Ornish, M.D., which demonstrated that the subjects affected changes in activity in about 500 genes—including 48 that were turned on and 453 genes that were turned off—as a result of eating more healthful foods, keeping stress levels down, practicing relaxation techniques such as meditation, and exercising regularly. Regarding the study, Dr. Ornish stated: "It's an exciting finding because so often people say, 'Oh, it's all in my genes, what can I do?' Well, it turns out you may be able to do a lot. In just three months, I can change hundreds of my genes simply by changing what I eat and how I live. That's pretty exciting."

Dr. Ornish's study demonstrates that we do indeed have control over our health by the choices we make. We just need to be better informed so that we can make those better choices. The present epidemic of overweight and obesity for most people is a result of a few choices made daily that, over time, have led to what's now the number one health crisis in this country. Optimal health is built on healthy *foundations*. It's the result of hundreds of choices you may make that gradually turn your well-being, at any given moment, toward its optimal level or toward disease. If a wise decision-making process isn't present, you'll still have some level of health—you'll still be alive—but you may be moving toward a disease state.

Remember that being vibrantly healthy results from decisions that you—and only you—can make. No one shoves poor food down your throat; you decide what to eat and how to live. Put another way, health isn't something you were born with that can't change, like your fingerprints. We all must take greater responsibility for our well-being. You can tell by your daily actions what you're committed to, what's a priority in your life. For example, do you say that you're committed to being healthy, but don't take time out to exercise and choose to eat healthful foods? Make your words count, and make vibrant health a top priority. Ralph Waldo Emerson would probably agree, since he said, "Health is our greatest wealth." How true that is!

Dan Chesnut, M.D., author of *Lying with Authority*, reinforces what Dr. Ornish's study shows. Dr. Chesnut states:

> Genes control everything in our body and they can cause disease when abnormal, but not always! So who controls genes? Nutrition can control genes. Genes can be silent and do nothing. Most are like that. For most genes to

become active (to be expressed) something in nutrition triggers it, bad or good. . . . Good genes that can boost immune activity can be expressed by good nutrition and that is good news. We know for sure that harmful genes can also be activated by animal products, especially cancer. That could be bad. . . . Weight gain may be influenced by 400 or more genes in worms! Probably in man, too. Plant-based nutrition beneficially affects gene activity. It can shut off or suppress "bad" genes. Animal-based food adversely affects gene activity. It can activate "bad" genes.

Consequences of Overweight and Obesity

Why does Dr. Fuhrman call obesity the number one health problem in America? Obesity and excess body weight is an underlying factor in a host of other disease conditions that significantly increase overall premature mortality. He states, "Obesity is not just a cosmetic issue—extra weight leads to an earlier death, as many studies confirm. Overweight individuals are more likely to die from all causes, including heart disease and cancer. Two-thirds of those with weight problems also have hypertension, diabetes, heart disease, or another obesity-related condition."

In the article, "The Hidden Dangers of Your Excess Abdominal Fat—More Than Just Vanity," which appeared on **www.IronMagazineForums.com**, Mike Geary, Certified Nutrition Specialist, Certified Personal Trainer, states:

What most people do not realize is that excess abdominal fat, in particular, is not only ugly, but is also a *dangerous risk factor to your health*. Scientific research has clearly demonstrated that although it is unhealthful in general to have excess body fat throughout your body, it is also particularly dangerous to have excess abdominal fat.

There are two types of fat that you have in your abdominal area. The first type that covers up your abs from being visible is called subcutaneous fat and lies directly beneath the skin and on top of the abdominal muscles.

The second type of fat that you have in your abdominal area is called visceral fat, and that lies deeper in the abdomen beneath your muscle and surrounding your organs. . . .

Both subcutaneous fat and visceral fat in the abdominal area are serious health risk factors, but science has shown that having excessive visceral fat is even more dangerous than subcutaneous fat. Both of them greatly increase your risk of developing heart disease, diabetes, high blood pressure, stroke, sleep apnea, various forms of cancer, and other degenerative diseases. [emphasis mine]

Research indicates that the entry of fats into the liver from abdominal stores may trigger increased insulin resistance which, in turn, may lead to diabetes. Our body uses insulin to open the door to the cells to allow the sugars circulating in the blood to be escorted into the cells to be used as energy. Circulating fats (especially animal fats and excess omega-6 fats) often cause the cells to be "resistant" to the efforts of insulin to escort the sugars into the cells. This "insulin resistance" signals the pancreas to produce more insulin in an effort to force the sugars into the cells. This becomes a vicious cycle that often leads to the use of drugs to help supply additional insulin. Unfortunately, all of the excess insulin leads to other problems, and the pancreas may become exhausted, leading to type 1 diabetes.

Fat tissue also is the storage site of many of the toxins the body is unable to eliminate. We live in an extremely toxic environment today. Our bodies are continually subjected to chemicals in our food, water, and air as well as from drugs that create a toxic load that often can't be eliminated efficiently. These toxins are stored in fat tissue until the body is equipped to deal with them. Our liver is designed to be a manufacturing and conversion facility as well as a detoxifier. It wasn't intended to deal with such an onslaught, so its ability to perform all of these tasks is limited. It's also called upon to deal with free-radical damage and the production and recycling of glutathione. This vital function is often hindered as the increasing toxic load takes precedence.

Leptin—an Essential Key in the Weight-Loss Struggle

In 1994, a key factor in weight loss was discovered. Jeffrey Friedman and colleagues at the Rockefeller University discovered the hormone leptin, which is produced by fat cells. Understanding the role of leptin in the body helps us understand why so many people struggle with weight loss and the inability to lose weight and keep it off long-term.

Leptin is produced by fat cells; interacts with six types of receptors; and helps regulate energy intake, energy expenditure, fat storage, and reproduction. The amount of fat determines, to a great extent, the amount of leptin that's produced.

At one time, scientists thought it was a deficiency of leptin that contributed to excess body weight, but now they've learned that it really isn't a *deficiency* but rather an *excess* of leptin that's compounding the problems in weight loss. Due to the excessive amount of the hormone that's produced by the fat cells, the neuron receptors have become *insensitive* to its signals. It's similar to being in a room where there's so much noise that you can't hear what someone's trying to say to you. With so much leptin circulating, the brain doesn't understand the signals to turn off the appetite, quit storing fat, and burn fat for energy.

Scientists at the University of Minnesota have invested seven years of research into a remarkable discovery about this hormone. They've learned that by reducing the amount of circulating leptin, sensitivity can be restored. Then the brain hears the signal to turn off the appetite and discontinue storing fat. As a result of this research, a composition supplement of polysaccharides was developed that helps reduce the production of leptin and restores sensitivity.

In an eight-week, double-blind, placebo-controlled study, scientists at the University of Connecticut Human Performance Laboratory demonstrated that when a sensible diet and moderate exercise were used along with a supplement known as *MaxWLX*—a weight-loss accelerator, the following results occurred. In eight weeks, the MaxWLX group lost 21.5 pounds of body fat, 3.96 inches off their waists, 3.28 inches off their hips, and 1.20 inches off each thigh. They achieved a 90 percent greater fat loss than the placebo group! (If you'd like to peruse the details of this exciting study, please go to: **www.WLXmovie.com**, **www.WLXvideo.com**, or **www.WLXstudy.com**.)

Time to Take Control

As I mentioned previously, excess weight carries many harmful implications and increases risk of diabetes. The hormones insulin and leptin may play critical roles in the inability of many people to shed the excess pounds and keep them off. While they truly may desire to take control of their health by adopting a healthful diet and lifestyle, the effect of a diet rich in refined sugar, refined grains, and processed foods can impair frontal-lobe function and the ability to make and follow wise choices long-term without some supplemental help.

In his book *Proof Positive,* Neil Nedley, M.D., explains the role of glucose as almost the exclusive source of energy for the brain. While the brain makes up about 2 percent of the body's mass, it accounts for about 15 percent of our total metabolism. When poor dietary factors require our body to produce an excess of insulin to deal with high levels of blood sugar, the extra insulin often causes too rapid a drop in blood sugar (a hypoglycemic response). This deprives the brain of the necessary glucose for normal mental function. Dr. Nedley tells us that it takes 45 to 75 minutes to regain standard intellectual function after the blood sugar returns to normal. With most people's reactive eating patterns, it's easy to see how they may lack the ability to make appropriate choices that would allow them to follow an optimal weight-loss program, especially when you factor in the role of leptin.

A well-balanced, natural-foods, plant-based diet—coupled with the stimulant-free, all-natural MaxWLX supplementation—can control the production of leptin and restore vital sensitivity to this hormone. Other beneficial factors include engaging in moderate exercise, keeping the body hydrated with an optimal intake of purified water, managing stress, and practicing relaxation techniques such as meditation or deep breathing. These lifestyle choices will enable most people to get the leptin production under control so their bodies aren't constantly being signaled to eat and store fats. An emphasis on plant-based foods will provide an abundance of nutrients with a lower caloric intake that promotes optimal insulin production and utilization. This, in turn, will allow for optimal mental function so that the shift can be a permanent change, not a temporary program.

By achieving an optimal body weight through healthful diet and lifestyle changes, the likelihood of developing diabetes and other chronic conditions is dramatically reduced. I challenge you today to choose the necessary steps that will allow you to take control of your health as well as your weight.

How to Get the Weight-Loss Accelerator

For more information on weight loss made easy and MaxWLX, please visit my Website: **www.SusanSmithJones.com** and click on "Maximize Health." There, you'll learn more about this revolutionary weight-loss accelerator (MaxWLX) and can order it for yourself and your loved ones. I encourage you to try it for three months. I've seen positive results from clients using it in my private practice as well as hearing success stories from countless others. If you'd like to order

MaxWLX today, along with two of my other favorite nutritional supplements —Max N•Fuze and the antiaging, anti-inflammatory, immune-boosting, detoxifying glutathione accelator, MaxGXL—please visit: **www.4HealthBliss.com** and click on "Products" for more information and "Preferred Customer" to receive wholesale pricing, as I do.

Another product that I highly recommend if you're interested in losing weight is Eng3's device, which helps your body use fat as its fuel source, enhancing weight loss. The device is totally natural, FDA approved, and can be combined with other treatments. You'll experience an acceleration of fat loss, especially if you adopt an optimal diet as described in my books and get regular exercise. (For more information, see Chapter 11.)

Finally, please refer to the first two books of this series, *The Healing Power of* Nature*Foods* and *Health Bliss*, and my other recent book, *Be Healthy~Stay Balanced,* for more detailed information on how to lose weight easily and effectively. This is one of the most requested topics when I do radio and TV interviews. On several occasions, people have told me that just these sections in the books are worth the cover price. You'll learn the best exercises to burn fat easily; the healthiest foods to accelerate fat loss; the most efficacious way to eat throughout the day to stoke your metabolism; the role of water to ramp up weight loss; which foods help your body burn *more* fat as a fuel source; and why you always want to nourish your spirit first before you can be successful at long-term weight loss and vibrant health. To order *The Healing Power of* Nature*Foods* and *Health Bliss*, please call: (800) 654-5126, or contact your local bookstore or **www.Amazon.com**.

I wish you vibrant health and a life free from weighty concerns forevermore.

CHAPTER 9

7 SUREFIRE STRESS BUSTERS

"Out of clutter, find simplicity. From discord, find harmony. In the middle of difficulty, lies opportunity."

— ALBERT EINSTEIN

Whether it's a new year, season, month, week, or day, you always can choose to make this moment a new beginning, opt to make choices about improving your health. One of the best ways to bring wellness into your world is to decrease the level of stress you experience on a daily basis. Why is this so important? Believe it or not, the American Association of Family Physicians reports that two-thirds of all doctor visits are due to stress-related ailments. It's also believed that 80 to 90 percent of all diseases are tied to tension. And if you're female, stress may be even more damaging to your health: study after study has found that women suffer from it and from depression more often than men.

For some of us, our biggest stressors might be weather-related situations such as tornados, earthquakes, floods, fires, or hurricanes. Similarly, most of us get anxious when thinking about deadlines and commitments, but stress has many other causes. It can be triggered by emotions—anger, fear, worry, grief, depression, or even guilt. And stress can actually lead to high blood pressure, heart problems, fatigue, muscle and joint pain, headaches, weight gain, and other illnesses and chronic health conditions. If you want to avoid these problems, follow my seven favorite tips to reduce stress, promote relaxation, and bring health and wellness to your body and world.

1. Get moving! Exercise is one of the best ways to reduce stress in your life because it relaxes muscles and eases tension. Want proof? A study at the University of Southern California showed that patients who took a vigorous walk and raised their heart rates to more than 100 beats per minute reduced the tension in their bodies by 20 percent. This effect was greater than a second group of patients who were given a tranquilizer! So go for a walk, hit the gym for some weight-bearing exercises, or give yoga a try. Studies have shown that those who practice yoga have lower stress hormones than those who don't.

2. Meditate and breathe deeply. Don't worry—you don't have to be a Buddhist monk to know how to meditate. Really, it's simple! Find a special, quiet space in your home. Spend at least 15 minutes here first thing in the morning and before going to bed. Sit and close your eyes and focus on your breathing. Inhale and exhale slowly and deeply, focusing on the sound and rhythm of your breathing. Mentally visualize peace and calmness. Your day will start and end on a stress-free note.

3. Eat a stress-relieving diet. Can your diet really help in this area? You bet. Take stress off your digestive system by getting at least seven servings of fresh fruits and vegetables daily. They're high in water content and easily digested. Especially beneficial are antioxidant-rich leafy greens, such as romaine lettuce, spinach, Swiss chard, kale, and collards. Choose an array of colors when it comes to produce in order to benefit from an array of antioxidants.

4. Keep your body hydrated. Our bodies are 70 percent water, our cells are 70 percent water, and our planet is 70 percent water. That's no coincidence. Each day we need to drink at least 8 glasses of water—even more (10 to 12) when it's hot, when we've been exercising, or in a dry climate or atmosphere such as in an airplane. At a cellular level, dehydration makes us as droopy as neglected violets. Lack of moisture in faces causes wrinkles the way lack of moisture in grapes causes raisins.

Drinking "liquids" won't do. Although herbal tea, freshly extracted vegetable juice, and diluted fruit juice can count in the water tally, coffee, tea, colas, and alcoholic beverages actually dehydrate the body. They're wet, but they're not water; in fact, they're *anti*-water.

We need to maintain proper fluid balance for brain and kidney function, to rid the body of waste material and toxins, and to maintain radiant health. Water is also a safe, cheap, and effective appetite suppressant. Often when we think we're hungry, we're actually thirsty. Get into the habit of carrying a bottle of water when you walk or drive. If it's there, you're more likely to drink it. You can refill it from your filtered or purified supply at home.

5. Catch plenty of Zzzs. Lack of sleep undermines your body's ability to deal with stress. That's why it's important to get eight hours of rest per night. One way to tell if you're getting enough shut-eye is to see if you wake at a regular time without an alarm. If you require a buzzer to get out of bed in the morning, you're not getting enough sleep.

6. Laugh a lot. Worried about something? Maybe you're stressed out about a relationship with a loved one, the monthly bills that are stacking up, or the poor

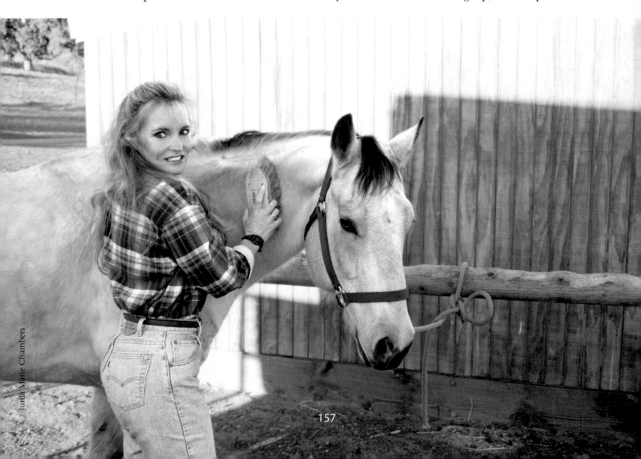

Jurita Marie Chambers

grades your son or daughter is suddenly bringing home from school. Whatever it is, one way to mollify this stress is to make sure your life is filled with laughter.

According to researchers, laughter releases endorphins into the body that act as natural stress beaters. In fact, a good belly laugh gives your heart muscles a workout; improves circulation; fills your lungs with oxygen-rich air; clears your respiratory passages; stimulates alertness hormones; helps relieve pain; and counteracts fear, anger, and depression, all of which are linked to illness and stress. So be sure to schedule time to be with friends and family members who make you smile and laugh, and go to movies or read a book that tickles your funny bone. Just make sure you're finding plenty of things to giggle about in your life.

7. Be thankful—and reap the health benefits. Each and every day, take a moment and be grateful for all you have in life. Gratitude, after all, is a great stress buster. What you think about consistently brings more of the same into your life. So focusing on the positive, even during difficult times, is the best way to reduce and alleviate stress and transform your life.

As you experiment with many of the recipes in this book, I hope that you'll also take heed of many of the lifestyle suggestions on how to create vibrant health that are sprinkled throughout.

"The whole course of things goes to teach us faith."

— Ralph Waldo Emerson

WATER: THE FOUNTAIN OF YOUTH & VITALITY

*"You can accomplish anything if you do not accept limitations
. . . whatever you make up your mind to do, you can do."*

— PARAMAHANSA YOGANANDA

Since our bodies are approximately 70 percent water, the key to a healthful lifestyle may be as simple as the water we drink every day. Water is one of the fundamental elements of life. Finding pure sources is essential in this modern era when environmental toxins abound. In ancient times, the cleanest water came from wells, streams, and rainwater. Now, after 100 years of high usage of chemicals and pesticides, well water, rivers, and rain are often polluted. Tap water is even worse because it's usually been treated with "cleansing" chemicals.

Plants have the natural ability to distill water. The method by which modern water purifiers remove unwanted chemicals and bacteria is very similar to that of a plant. Filters range from eliminating only odor and taste to removing all unwanted inorganic minerals and harmful bacteria. Water distillers evaporate the water and recondense it, leaving toxic sediment behind. Reverse osmosis (a filtering process) also purifies water, rendering it much healthier than tap water. However, in my estimation, the best device is an ionizer, which I'll discuss at the end of this section.

In addition to transporting vital nutrients, water regulates the body's temperature; allows for easier digestion; lubricates the joints; helps eliminate wastes;

WATER: THE FOUNTAIN OF YOUTH & VITALITY

*"You can accomplish anything if you do not accept limitations
. . . whatever you make up your mind to do, you can do."*

— PARAMAHANSA YOGANANDA

Since our bodies are approximately 70 percent water, the key to a healthful lifestyle may be as simple as the water we drink every day. Water is one of the fundamental elements of life. Finding pure sources is essential in this modern era when environmental toxins abound. In ancient times, the cleanest water came from wells, streams, and rainwater. Now, after 100 years of high usage of chemicals and pesticides, well water, rivers, and rain are often polluted. Tap water is even worse because it's usually been treated with "cleansing" chemicals.

Plants have the natural ability to distill water. The method by which modern water purifiers remove unwanted chemicals and bacteria is very similar to that of a plant. Filters range from eliminating only odor and taste to removing all unwanted inorganic minerals and harmful bacteria. Water distillers evaporate the water and recondense it, leaving toxic sediment behind. Reverse osmosis (a filtering process) also purifies water, rendering it much healthier than tap water. However, in my estimation, the best device is an ionizer, which I'll discuss at the end of this section.

In addition to transporting vital nutrients, water regulates the body's temperature; allows for easier digestion; lubricates the joints; helps eliminate wastes;

and keeps skin healthy, youthful, and attractive. Not drinking enough water can lead to dehydration, which may result in frequent headaches, general fatigue, dizziness, constipation, and impaired memory and vision. A shortage of water also will result in excess weight, because too little of this element causes our bodies to store water outside of our cells, making us feel bloated and heavy.

Drinking plenty of water will help you lose or maintain a healthful weight. It's calorie free, suppresses the appetite naturally, and helps metabolize fat. Without enough water, your kidneys can't function properly, which forces them to send some of their workload to your liver. Since one of that organ's main functions is to metabolize stored fat, the added work from the kidneys means that the liver burns less fat so that more remains on the body—usually on the waist, hips, and thighs. If you're overweight, it's a good idea to drink at least three extra glasses of water daily over the recommended eight.

It's just too expensive to purchase all of your water in plastic bottles from the store; besides, you want to reduce your use of noxious plastic containers. I encourage everyone to check out the Ionizer Plus®, which is the home machine that I've used and recommended for more than 15 years. Through a process of electrolysis, this superlative device concentrates minerals (calcium, magnesium, and potassium) already present in your water. In the process of doing so, the minerals get split into the highly bioavailable ionic form, and the resulting water is alkaline (it has a pH greater than 7.0). The electrolysis also reduces the surface tension of the water, making it more easily absorbed by the body.

As you alkalinize your body, you maximize your health. This advanced Ionizer Plus first filters the tap water to remove contaminants, chlorine, chemicals, and foul taste. Next, it enters an electrolysis chamber, which divides it into Alkali-ion and Acidic-ion water. The reduced molecular clusters permeate the body quickly and efficiently. This device is paramount in my health program. I use the machine's alkaline water for drinking and meal preparation and the acid water for my skin and plants. For more information, visit my Website, **www.SusanSmithJones.**

com and click on "Susan's Favorite Products." To order an Ionizer Plus, visit: **www.hightechhealth.com** or call: 800-794-5355.

In at least two of my daily glasses of water from my Ionizer Plus, I add a couple of tablespoons of one of my favorite salubrious health supplements called E3Live. This is one of nature's most perfect superfoods, and the world's first and only fresh-frozen live Aphanizomenon flos-aquae (AFA). Here's a brief background: For thousands of years, algae have been used worldwide as an excellent food source and potent medicine. For 25 years, the naturally occurring AFA growing in Klamath Lake, Oregon, has been harvested and sold as a unique dietary supplement that's extremely nutrient rich. It provides more chlorophyll than wheatgrass; it's 60 percent high-quality protein; it has all of the B vitamins, including B_{12}; it provides essential omega-3 and omega-6 fatty acids; and it's teeming with powerful digestive enzymes. This is the only AFA product that's organic, kosher, vegan, raw—and so versatile.

For more than 12 years, it's been a staple in my diet and a healthful food I recommend to everyone. This delicious green liquid (various flavors are available) can be combined with water, added to juices or smoothies, or simply enjoyed by the tablespoon. I encourage you to try it for 90 days—just one season—and see all of the positive effects it will have on your physical, mental, emotional, and spiritual well-being. You'll find information on E3Live on my Website when you click on "Susan's Favorite Products." Ask the company Vision, the harvesters of E3Live, to send you their excellent free CD. It beautifully describes the product and what it can do for your hair, skin, body, and overall well-being. For more detailed information or to order, please visit: **www.E3Live.com** or call: (888) 800-7070 or (541) 273-2212.

Now drink up, and as you do, remember to celebrate yourself and life.

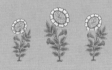

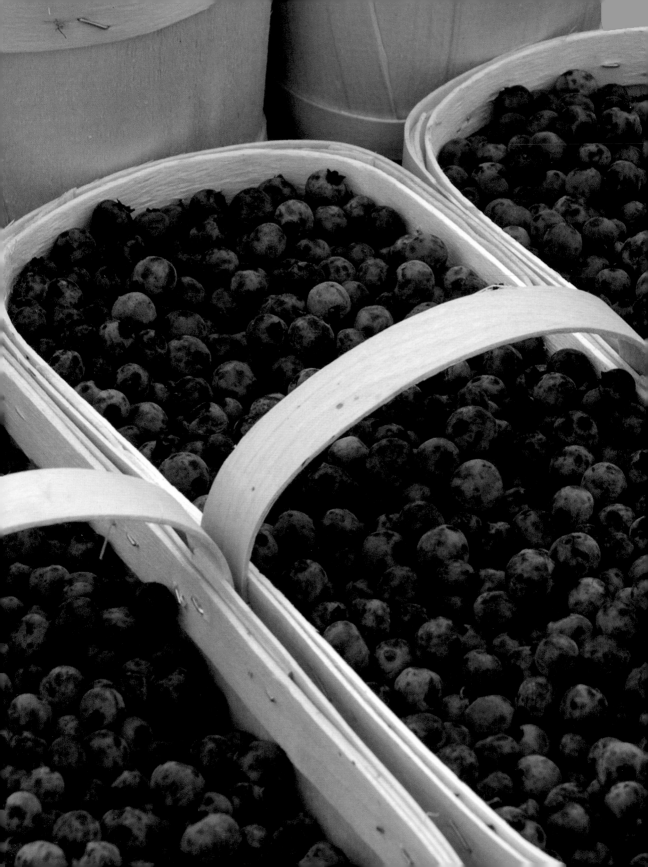

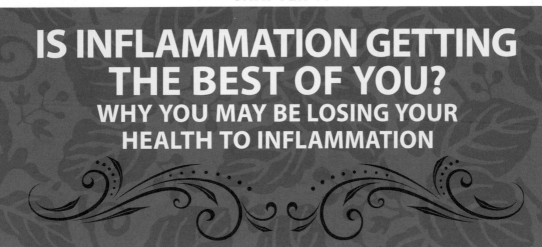

CHAPTER 11

IS INFLAMMATION GETTING THE BEST OF YOU?
WHY YOU MAY BE LOSING YOUR HEALTH TO INFLAMMATION

"No one can make you feel inferior without your consent."

— ELEANOR ROOSEVELT

Most of us never give a second thought to inflammation unless we are stung by a bee, experience a physical injury such as stubbing our toes on a piece of furniture, or injure our backs. As soon as one of these events takes place, we experience an immediate sensation of pain that tells us something is definitely wrong. Redness, heat, and swelling usually follow. This reaction is a result of inflammation. Unfortunately, the most devastating diseases known to humankind—including cancer, heart disease, diabetes, asthma, Parkinson's, and Alzheimer's—are almost always preceded by months and years of very subtle, unnoticed inflammation.

Inflammation can be good in that often the swelling and pain limit the range of motion for an injured body part, allowing it to heal. However, when subtle inflammation continues for too long, it becomes destructive. Almost all diseases are preceded and accompanied by this physical reaction. In this chapter, I'll explore what's involved with inflammation, its impact on the body, what we can do to reduce uncontrolled inflammation and its damaging effects on our health, and how to preclude falling prey to misleading nutritional information.

In his book *Inflammation Nation*, Floyd H. Chilton, Ph.D., provides some interesting insights. He discusses inflammation in the sense of it being a "double-edged sword"—both a helper and a villain. While it's great when it serves as a warning signal (as in the stubbed-toe example), it becomes a villain when initiated by diet and lifestyle, subtly beginning an uncontrolled destructive process in the body that goes unnoticed for decades until a disease appears. Dr. Chilton states:

> We are unquestionably facing an epidemic in inflammatory disease. By my estimate, approximately half of all Americans suffer from an inflammatory disorder, and even more of us are at risk.
>
> By contrast (contrasting the infectious diseases of the previous century that have been almost entirely eradicated with inflammatory diseases of today), non-infectious inflammatory diseases have gotten worse in each of the last three decades. A physician friend of mine jokes that Celebrex has replaced Prozac as the "must-have" drug of the decade.
>
> A silent plague is sweeping America, and the vast majority of us are at risk.

Dan Chesnut, M.D., explains in his book *Lying with Authority:*

> Inflammation results when cells are sick, traumatized, chemically irritated, infected, etc. Sick zones always signal the immune system for assistance. It is important to realize that inflammation can occur in a low-grade, barely noticeable way, especially in the brain. Almost all vaccines can cause brain inflammation, which may last for as long as a year. Even stress and depression can cause a low-grade, unnoticed inflammation and signals are sent to the immune system for help.
>
> When immune cells or other immune components rush into sick or "hot" zones, *free radicals* are formed during the heat of battle. . . . Free radicals can be released and always have the potential of cell and DNA damage, which can lead to disease.

Left unchecked, these free radicals can damage a cell membrane or, when created within a cell, hurt the DNA. The body has a built-in system for dealing with and preventing free-radical damage when all cells are functioning optimally. But when they aren't, problems arise.

Those Pesky Free Radicals

A diet rich in antioxidants provides "free-radical scavengers" that neutralize these compounds before damage occurs and, ideally, also should supply raw materials from which each individual cell can produce its own master antioxidant, glutathione (also known as GSH), which I'll discuss later. Unfortunately, today our diet of nutritionally deficient foods doesn't support our bodies' efforts to prevent free-radical damage. Our cells are malnourished and toxins aren't eliminated efficiently. As a result, they're becoming sicker by the day.

Prolonged tissue inflammation caused by tobacco smoke, alcohol abuse, chemical exposure, exposure to electromagnetic radiation, and improper diet produces a continuous onslaught of free radical damage that, left unchecked for years, often leads to various types of cancers. The February 2005 issue of *The Blaylock Wellness Report* stated:

> A recent study found that one central event is most closely associated with cancer development—chronic inflammation. In the study, researchers looked at a large number of cancer patients and found that almost 70 percent had preexisting chronic inflammatory diseases for 10 to 17 years *before* they developed cancer.
>
> We know that people with chronic inflammatory diseases like lupus and rheumatoid arthritis, as well as those with inflammatory bowel disease (Crohn's and ulcerative colitis) and certain parasitic diseases, have substantially higher cancer rates than that of normal people. If we include diabetes (also an inflammatory disease), we see that a great number of people are at risk.

In the June 2008 issue, Dr. Blaylock explained:

> It turns out that two physiological processes play a major role in inflammation: the immune system and the prostaglandin system. They interact with each other and either enhance inflammation—or reduce it.
>
> Now there is growing evidence that one or both of these systems stop functioning correctly in many people and get stuck in the inflammation mode. A process meant to speed recovery, in fact, goes into overdrive, causing potentially far greater problems.

Dr. Blaylock goes on to state that the key players that influence this process are toxins, infections, injury, and heredity, and that our diet has a major influence on all of these factors. Dr. Chilton is in full agreement: "I believe that our diet is a major—if not the most important—external factor behind the inflammation epidemic."

For more than a century, science has thought that certain chemical exposures, viruses, and even parasites can cause cancer and other chronic diseases. But are these the actual causes? Growing evidence seems to suggest that it is our body's natural *reactions* to these exposures that are behind it all.

Inflammation & Cancer

A wide variety of environmental and dietary exposures (such as pesticides, petroleum-based products, and animal products) long have been considered to be carcinogenic. Those suffering with diabetes, depression, and cardiovascular and autoimmune diseases generally have a higher risk of developing cancer. These conditions have one significant thing in common—they all cause inflammation, which itself may be a cause of subsequent disease. In this model, the inflammatory process may be a vicious cycle that's out of control!

Researchers are discovering that cancer often appears 15 to 17 years after the onset of inflammatory disease. One study found that 65 percent of whites and 70 percent of blacks suffered from prolonged inflammatory disease before developing cancer (Blaylock, June 2008). Ongoing inflammation also makes the cancers grow faster and spread more readily.

Since many processed foods are sources of inflammatory agents, which are found in additives, it's imperative that you avoid such products as much as possible. A diet of primarily raw, plant-based foods is most ideal and is anti-inflammatory.

Your diet and lifestyle are the foundation that support your body's efforts to maintain optimal health. The standard American diet (SAD) is rich in trans fats from partially hydrogenated oils, sugars, animal foods that promote inflammation, and the like. The SAD of today has about 50 times as much omega-6 fat as our ancestors consumed a century ago, and it's radically deficient in omega-3 fats. Excess omega-6 promotes inflammation, while omega-3 is anti-inflammatory. A plant-based diet with a high percentage of raw foods and a heavy emphasis on leafy green vegetables and omega-3-rich foods (such as flaxseed, walnuts, and flax oil) is anti-inflammatory and supports optimal health at the cellular level.

Life at the Cellular Level

Health is maintained at the cellular level. The vitality of each individual cell is critical in maintaining a body that's free of inflammation and disease. Each one must be able to take in nutrition, eliminate toxins efficiently, and replicate new healthy cells if our organs, tissues, and body are to maintain the highest level of health.

The normal processes of metabolism that take place on a daily basis, as we saw earlier, produce free radicals (oxidative stress) that the body must be able to deal with. Each individual cell is a small factory that carries out a multitude of actions on a continual basis. One of those very important functions is for the mitochondria to create energy through the production of adenosine triphosphate (ATP). This process also creates free radicals that, if not neutralized, may damage the cell membrane, the cellular DNA, or other areas of the cell. Fortunately, the body has a built-in mechanism to handle this damage when all is functioning optimally.

The Master Antioxidant—Glutathione

Unfortunately, however, everything isn't functioning optimally for most people, and their level of health is on a gradual decline. Each cell produces glutathione (GSH)—the "master antioxidant"—when it has the necessary raw materials. The intracellular glutathione has the ability to neutralize the free radical damage that results from the mitochondria's production of ATP (energy). Glutathione is capable of neutralizing thousands of free radicals while antioxidants such as vitamin C and vitamin E only take care of a very limited number. The antioxidant activity of both vitamins is supported by glutathione in much the same way.

In *GSH: Your Body's Most Powerful Protector Glutathione,* Jimmy Gutman, M.D., FACEP, discussed vitamin C's role as an antioxidant:

When a vitamin C molecule mops up a free radical, it effectively neutralizes it. However, the vitamin C complex is now tied up. It is either ejected from the cell and eliminated by the body, or it is recycled to go back and do more work. In the latter case, glutathione is the recycling agent; GSH and GSH enzymes accept the free radical from the vitamin C complex and free it up to get back to work. This cycle drives antioxidant function in our bodies.

Researchers have learned that beyond the age of 20, the body's ability to produce glutathione declines by 10 to 12 percent per decade. It's thought that this decline is related to poor diet and lifestyle, as well as other external influences on the body. The raw materials necessary for the production of glutathione are often lacking in the diet. And unfortunately, this antioxidant isn't a supplement that can be taken with any significant benefit, as orally ingested glutathione is degraded in the stomach environment and never reaches the cellular level where it is critically needed.

Dr. Gutman states:

> Blood-GSH concentrations in younger people (20–40 years) have been shown to be some 20–40 percent higher than in older people (60–80 years). Studies by some of the world's leading experts on aging suggest that elderly individuals with elevated GSH levels have a physical advantage over those with lower levels. Those with 20 percent higher blood levels have been found to experience approximately one-third the rate of arthritis, high blood pressure, heart disease, circulatory difficulties, and other various maladies than others.

Glutathione & Vibrant Health

One common characteristic seen in patients diagnosed with asthma, Parkinson's, Alzheimer's, AIDS, multiple sclerosis, cancer, and a host of other diseases is that they're all usually dramatically low in glutathione. Low levels of intracellular glutathione mean that free radicals are neutralized less efficiently, and inflammation goes on uncontrolled.

In the *Encyclopedia of Natural Medicine*, author and nutrition researcher Michael Murray, N.D., talks about glutathione's role as a master antioxidant and detoxifier:

This combination of detoxification and protection from free radicals results in glutathione being one of the most important anticarcinogens and antioxidants in our cells, which means a deficiency is devastating. When we are exposed to high levels of toxins, glutathione is used up faster than it can be produced or absorbed from the diet. We then become much more susceptible to toxin-induced diseases such as cancer, especially if our phase one detoxification system is highly active. Diseases that result from glutathione deficiency are not uncommon. A deficiency can be induced by diseases that increase the need for glutathione, deficiencies of the nutrients needed for glutathione synthesis, or diseases that inhibit the formation of glutathione

Dr. Robert Keller, M.D.—chairman, CEO, CSO of Phoenix BioSciences—and practicing physician, is considered to be one of the greatest scholars of the 21st century. Dr. Keller believes the decrease in production of glutathione is much more rapid than stated in scientific literature. He attributes much of this decline to lack of nutrition and the extensive toxic load our bodies are subjected to from our environment, water, food, and lifestyles.

These factors have a negative impact on the ability of each individual cell to produce energy, eliminate waste, and function optimally. The immune system is then impaired, and the body's innate ability to self-heal can't function as designed. "The protective activity of GSH is twofold: It enhances the activity of the immune cells and also functions as an antioxidant within them," Dr. Gutman says.

In his medical practice, Dr. Keller has found that almost all of his critically ill patients have had one thing in common—they were dramatically low in glutathione. During more than a decade of intensive research on glutathione's role in the body, he's found a way to increase the glutathione levels in his patients so that they can enjoy a greater quality of life. Interestingly, Dr. Keller notes that individuals who live to the age of 100 have the GSH levels of a 40-year-old. This is indicative of the protection that higher levels of glutathione afford an individual as he or she ages!

The Best Form of Glutathione

If you think that all you need to do is visit your local pharmacy or natural-food store to purchase a bottle of glutathione, think again. As I mentioned, it can't be used in supplemental form with any significant benefit; when the protein molecule is broken down in the stomach, it's degraded so much that it's no longer GSH. Until Dr. Keller's recent, cutting-edge discovery, the most efficient way of increasing glutathione levels was by injection. Not only is this a merely short-term solution, but it's also quite expensive.

After more than ten years of trial and error, Dr. Keller learned how to combine the building blocks of GSH in such a way that they could make it much easier for the body to produce more optimal intracellular levels of GSH.

Now, thanks to him, we have available a simple, inexpensive, and scientifically proven way to improve our ability to produce glutathione (GSH) at the cellular level by *300 percent and more over a three-month period of time.* In speaking of Dr. Keller's discovery, John Nelson, M.D., MPH, FACOG, and past president of the American Medical Association stated: "This product, in my opinion, represents the single most important breakthrough in health that I will witness in my lifetime. I believe it will revolutionize, change, and transform the practice of medicine worldwide and make Dr. Robert Keller more famous than Jonas Salk, who created the polio vaccine."

To learn more about Dr. Keller and his amazing glutathione accelerator (MaxGXL), please visit: **www.4HealthBliss.com**, click on his picture and listen to his interview. Additionally, you'll also enjoy listening to another interview on glutathione and vibrant health here: **weeu.com/mp3/idol51208.mp3**. Finally, you also may want to visit **www.SusanSmithJones.com**, click on "Maximize Health," and peruse the variety of information I've included on glutathione and why it's such a stellar supplement.

Susan's Personal Favorite

On a personal note, I've been taking Dr. Keller's nutritional supplement for some time now, and it has made a profound difference in how I feel and look. I now have more energy, recover faster after workouts; sleep more easily and deeply; and even experience better concentration, focus, and mental alertness from taking this supplement.

Some of the clients in my private practice have experienced much easier weight loss and noticeable relief from PMS, menopause symptoms, muscle and joint pain, fibromyalgia, fatigue, diabetes, colds and flu, cellular inflammation, accelerated aging, cardiovascular disease, and so much more. I encourage you to try it for three months and see how much better you look and feel.

When optimal levels of GSH are available, a person often experiences renewed energy as well as vibrant health and youthful vitality. Because most of us live in an environment where not only are many of our foods toxic from chemicals and environmental pollution, but our water and air are also polluted, it has become increasingly important to supplement our diet with nutrients that support optimum health. MaxGXL is that supplement.

For more information or to order, please visit: **www.4HealthBliss.com**. If you'd like to get wholesale pricing, as I do, then click on "Preferred Customer" to order easily and quickly as you also register for regular monthly shipments to keep you continually supplied with this remarkable product, which you won't want to be without. You'll thank your lucky stars that you found out about this cutting-edge, breakthrough compound and are making it part of your daily health regimen. I wouldn't do without this salubrious supplement.

Enhanced Oxygen Utilization

Another product that I highly recommend is a device from Eng3 that helps you get the most from the nutrients you ingest because of the oxygen utilization. It reduces inflammation and helps your body use fat as its fuel source, which enhances weight loss. The device is totally natural and contains no chemicals or drugs of any kind. It's completely safe, FDA approved, and can be combined with other treatments.

As we age, our cells lose the ability to effectively use the oxygen in the air we breathe, even if we practice deep breathing on a regular basis. Eng3's device helps you to optimize your oxygen supply and maximize the ability of your cells to produce energy (ATP), which is the best protection against illness and the effects of aging. Optimized cellular energy production improves overall health and quality of life, retards age-related diseases and disorders, reduces damage from excess free radicals, enhances cellular regeneration, maximizes our ability to draw nutrition from the food we eat, improves athletic performance, and shortens recovery time.

I've been using the device for years; and I've seen noticeable, positive differences in how I look and feel. My clients love it, too. I now sleep better, have an easier time concentrating and focusing on my work, exercise harder without tiring, recover more rapidly, and have more energy than I ever dreamed possible. All of these benefits come from using it for just 20 minutes per day, three days per week. I use it when watching TV, working at my computer, and meditating. Some of my clients even enjoy it when sleeping.

If you're interested in losing weight and restoring youthful vitality, definitely consider purchasing this product. You'll experience an acceleration of fat loss, especially if you adopt an optimal diet (as described in my books) and get regular exercise. To order or to find out if this device is for you, simply visit: **www.Eng3corp.com** or call: (877) 571-9206. They'll be happy to answer all of your questions. A healthier, happier, and more energized life could be just a few breaths away.

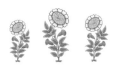

CHAPTER 12

SPROUTING YOUR WAY TO VIBRANCY

"Any religion which is not based on a respect for life is not a true religion."

— ALBERT SCHWEITZER

n his glorious poetry collection entitled *Leaves of Grass*, Walt Whitman wrote: "The smallest sprout shows there is really no death." As a food, sprouts are approximately 5,000 years old. In 2939 B.C., the emperor of China wrote about their versatile qualities, and these little gems still remain one of the most nutritious foods on earth. The humble sprout truly is one of nature's most amazing creations.

If you believe in eating a living-foods diet, then you're probably well acquainted with sprouts. These remarkable gifts of nature are pure, fresh, nutrient-rich, and alive with their vital force intact. If you're interested in experiencing healing, optimal health, and vitality, then make sprouts—the food for the future—part of your salubrious kitchen and lifestyle. Sprouts have been a cornerstone of my wellness program for the past 35 years. Think about it this way: What food can you easily produce and enjoy whether you're 3 years old or 103, vegan or carnivore, while living in an inner-city high-rise or on an isolated island? What's grown indoors with no soil, is harvested in two to seven days, and is loved by children and adults alike? What can supply your family with fresh vegetables year-round, regardless of the season? What food is edible raw or cooked, and is delicious either eaten all by itself or included in an exciting array of recipes?

The answer is *sprouts*.

Nature's Little Miracle

Start with a small, dry, hard seed. Add warm air and a little water, and watch as new life emerges as if by magic from the dormant seed. Vibrant with life and bursting with energy, its tiny size belies the extraordinary activity that takes place while growing. In mere hours and at a cost to you of just pennies, its delicate shoot proceeds to provide the most vital food imaginable.

Sprouts increase in nutritional content as they grow, and this increase proves to be truly remarkable. The vitamin C in sprouted peas increases eightfold in four days. In four days of sprouting, the vitamin B complex in sprouted wheat increases sixfold, and vitamin E increases threefold. Increased nutritional value doesn't stop there. Many different minerals abound in sprouts, and in an assimilable form. These little treasures provide a storehouse of enzymes; and all vegetables, nuts, seeds, beans, and grains begin life as sprouts.

Homegrown sprouts are the freshest, most assuredly organic food available to you. Nothing compares with "picking your own" just before you eat them and knowing they're free from fungicides and insecticides. When you eat sprouts, you're receiving the plant's peak nutrition, when nature has mobilized all of its nourishment to bring forth a mature plant.

Try this experiment: Assuming that almonds and sunflower seeds are already "delish" to your taste buds, soak them in filtered water for half a day, drain, and eat them as they are. If you agree that simply soaking improves their taste and digestibility, welcome to your new life as a gardener and sprout gourmet. Grains, beans, and seeds are easy to sprout and delectable to eat. They range in shape and color from the concave lens of the brown lentil to the oval of the golden alfalfa seed. Many know of mung-bean sprouts from Chinese restaurants, but how about sprouted rice?

In a simple glass jar that requires neither sunlight nor soil, and with only an hour's work spread over three days, you can cultivate more than 30 varieties of sprouts. You don't need to toil long and hard, sweating under the summer and fall sun, defending your crop from insects and weeds. Yet you're fully assured that your harvest is organically grown, absolutely fresh, and resoundingly cheap. And if you don't have the desire or inclination to do your own sprouting in the comfort of your kitchen, you can find freshly grown sprouts in most natural-food stores as well as many supermarkets.

Botanically speaking, all nuts, grains, and beans are seeds of plants. Every seed can create a new plant, which creates a thousand new seeds, which produce whole fields and forests. This occurs naturally enough in nature, but to imitate this process in your kitchen, you must learn to control the air, water, darkness, and warmth necessary for successful germination.

Let's Get Started

You need a few simple things—a container; air; water; darkness; warmth; and seeds, grains, or beans. Almost any container that permits drainage can serve as a sprouting vessel, including earthenware crocks, flower pots, bamboo trays, natural or nylon cloth bags, commercial sprouting trays and kits, and colanders. Make sure that the container isn't made of aluminum or any metal prone to rust. The one that I use—the most suitable and the simplest—is a wide-mouth glass jar. Most natural-food and high-end kitchen stores carry some kind of sprout container. You even can recycle empty glass jars from mayonnaise, nut butters, and canning, but be sure to use a wide-mouth quart (or liter) jar and not the small pints or narrow-mouth quarts.

Whatever jar or container you choose, it must be rendered drainable. You can perforate the metal cap by punching holes with an ice pick or hammering holes with a nail. The caps will soon rust unless occasionally lubricated with your favorite salad oil. Instead of the metal cap, I've used cotton muslin, cheesecloth, and even a fine wire mesh that I secure on the rim of the jar with a rubber band.

Homemade mesh sprout tops for mason jars are not only economical, they're also easy to make and use. Remove the lids of the jar caps and retain the rings. Purchase from the hardware store a small section of nylon, copper, or non-galvanized window screen. Use the lids as patterns for cutting circles out of the screen, and insert these screen circles back into the rings instead of the lids. As with metal jar caps, the metal rings eventually rust. By then you will qualify as an experienced sprouter, at which time you may feel commercial sprout tops are a worthy investment.

Sold in health-food stores, commercial tops fit wide-mouth jars. The more widely available tops are all plastic, while the super deluxe models consist of plastic rings with removable stainless steel screens. Both models come in different meshes, each appropriate for the individual stages and species of sprouts. For instance, the fine mesh is perfect for one-day-old alfalfa sprouts or any-day-old bean sprouts.

Sprouts are very hearty and can survive less than pristine conditions. If your tap water is heavily chlorinated, however, set it in an open container for one day or boil it for one minute. The chlorine will dissipate. Personally, I'm glad that I have a stellar water-filtration system that guarantees I'm using only the best ionized water with a pH of around 9.5 for growing my sprouts and hydrating my body. (If you visit **www.SusanSmithJones.com** and click on "Susan's Favorite Products," you can learn more about my favorite water purifier and filtration system: Ionizer Plus.)

Room temperature is a crucial factor in determining the growth rate of your sprouts. It also affects how often you need to rinse them. For instance, three rinses a day for two summer days yields the same growth as two rinses a day for three winter days. The desirable rinsing frequency depends upon room temperature. If it's too cold, sprout near a radiator, heating vent, or fish tank, or in the warmest room of your home.

Purchasing the Best Seeds, Grains & Beans

Where should you purchase your seeds, grains, and beans for sprouting? Regular supermarkets sell a few whole seeds and grains, but their whole beans are often irradiated or chemically treated to inhibit sprouting. If you try them, you're likely to concoct only a soupy slime. Dead or dying beans may be low quality for sprouting, but they're still food, so neither despair nor discard them. Cook them into soup— which is exactly what they're sold for.

Garden seeds are dependably viable, but seldom edible. Seeds intended for planting are treated with fungicides and insecticides, which, if eaten in large quantities, can make you very sick or may even be fatal. And untreated garden seeds, measured by the ounce, are prohibitively priced.

The most reliable sources of viable seeds are health-food stores and mail-order distribution. Among the latter, some even specialize in seeds for sprouting. When I'm sampling any new seed source, I always buy a small quantity, and I always buy organic. You might locate a bulk mail-order bargain price for five pounds of sunflower seeds, but if they sprout poorly, then you've bought expensive birdseed. Never stock more than you'll need until the next fall harvest. That five-pound sack of sunflower seeds is no bargain if it lasts two years. Germination rates decrease every year, particularly every summer. The identical air, warmth, and light that cause soaked seeds to sprout in a very short time also cause stored seeds to deteriorate over a very long time.

Always store unhulled seeds, whole grains, and dry beans in the dark and away from heat. Refrigerate hulled sunflower and pumpkin seeds and shelled almonds and peanuts. Store in airtight, preferably glass, containers. Most (but not all) plastic containers affect the smell of the air just as they do the taste of water. Particularly avoid plastic bags because they do a poor job of keeping insects either out or in.

An Easy Process

The process of sprouting is really quite simple. As an example, I'll explain how to sprout alfalfa seeds since most people know what alfalfa sprouts are and like them.

Measure two tablespoons of seeds. Discard any stones, twigs, or other foreign matter that might be in with the seeds. Place the measured and culled seeds into the jar, then fill it three-quarters full with room-temperature water. Swirl the jar vigorously, or stir the seeds with a long wooden spoon. Pour off the UFOs (the Unidentified Floating Objects). Some seeds may float to the top. These may be infertile, and I usually discard them. Drain and fill the jar with water again, repeating this step until the water appears clear and the surface is free of UFOs. After the last clean drain, fill the jar one more time and cover with a screen top—because air ventilation is important even at this submerged stage.

Alfalfa or clover (my favorite) should soak from three to eight hours, depending upon the room temperature; the warmer it is, the shorter the soak time.

For other seeds, soaking times vary. A common denominator is eight hours or overnight: a one-night stand! Let the seeds stand in the water while you're sleeping—your sprouts will be waking.

To drain the soaking water efficiently, select the proper size screen for the jar top. Choose the widest mesh for maximum ventilation and drainage, but not so wide that you throw out the baby seeds with the bath water. For alfalfa, start with your finest mesh for the first two days, switch to a medium mesh for the third and fourth days, and graduate to the widest mesh for the fifth and sixth days.

Soaking water is rich in water-soluble vitamins and minerals, so don't pour it down the kitchen sink. While bean water is unfit for consumption, if you wish to remain sociable and comfortably silent, grain and seed waters are ideal ingredients in soups and sauces. Refrigerate what you don't use immediately or else it will ferment into a near beer. You can also feed all excess bean, grain, and seed water to your house or garden plants.

After draining the soaking water, rinse the seeds, always using room-temperature water. Cold will shock the sprouts; hot will kill them. To rinse, run the water along the walls inside the jar (not directly onto the sprouts), and fill nearly to capacity. Dislodge any seeds that stick high on the walls by gently twirling the jar. Allow the seeds to remain submerged for a few moments, and then pour off the water. I always lean the jar against the side of the sink (in my dish drainer) to drip there for five minutes. And because water will continually collect at the bottom of the jar, you *must* devise a setup to keep the jar inverted at a slight angle until the next rinse, 8 to 10 hours later. If you lay the jar flat, a puddle will gather inside, leading to rot, which causes crop failure.

Small seeds, such as alfalfa and clover, require twice-a-day rinsing. Large beans dry out easily, so they need to be rinsed more often—four or more times a day. Don't worry! After a couple weeks of sprouting, you'll be able to do this in your sleep—well, almost. The routine will become habitual and even enjoyable. I love seeing the seeds and beans magically turn into edible, nutritious, and delicious food.

Sunning and Rinsing

On the fourth or fifth day, expose your now-leafy alfalfa to indirect sunlight. Avoid doing so before the third day, or the sprouts will dry out from the heat of even indirect sunlight. Leafy sprouts, such as alfalfa, clover, broccoli, cabbage, kale, radish, spinach, mustard, and turnip—as well as the more difficult chia, cress, and flax—all grow leaves. And all leaves will eventually develop chlorophyll when exposed to light. Sometimes all you need is a single day of indirect sun.

When your sprouts are fully grown, transfer them into a bowl filled with water. Place the bowl in the sink in order to accommodate overflow and spills. Loosen the clumps of sprouts from each other—you're combing out the hulls. Gently agitate and submerge the sprouts with one hand and let the hulls float to the top or sink to the bottom. I remove the hulls and repeat as necessary. This entire process, which may seem complicated when reading, is really easy to do.

After the sprouts are drained well, refrigerate them. (But never refrigerate sprouts that are dripping wet from the most recent rinsing because they'll turn mushy after one to two days.) Thoroughly wash and dry the sprouting jar between each batch.

At this point, soak some more seeds. I have several stages of sprout jars going in my kitchen all of the time, so I'm never without delicious sprouts to eat out of hand or add to my favorite recipes. Tending sprouts should be a joy, not a chore. Grow them, knowing that you're being good to them; and thank them, knowing they'll be good for you.

Sprouting Guide

For your convenience, here's a Sprouting Guide so that you'll know the particulars for soaking, rinsing, harvesting, and special uses for all kinds of seeds, grains, and beans.

	Soaking time in hours	Number of times to rinse and drain per day	Average number of days until harvest	Special handling
Alfalfa/Clover	8	3	3–4	None
Beets	8	3	3–5	None
Buckwheat	8	3	2–3	Remove remaining husks
Chia	8	0	3–5	Mist gently with water 3 times a day
Corn	8	3	2–4	None
Cress	0	0	3–5	Mist gently with water 3 times a day
Dill	8	3	3–5	None
Fenugreek	8	3	3–5	Mist gently with water 3 times a day
Flax	0	0	3–5	Mist gently with water 3 times a day
Garbanzo	8	3	3–4	None
Lentil	8	3	2–4	None
Millet	8	3	3–5	None
Mung Bean	8	3	3–4	None
Mustard	0	3	3–5	Mist gently with water 3 times a day
Napa Cabbage	8	3	3–4	None
Oats	8	3	2–3	Remove remaining husks
Peas	8	3	3–4	None
Radish	8	3	3–4	None
Red Clover	8	3	3–5	None
Rye	8	3	2–3	None
Sesame	8	3	2–3	None
Soybean	24	3	3–5	Change soaking water every 8 hours
Sunflower	8	3	3–5	Remove remaining husks
Wheat	8	3	2	None

You can use the various sprouts in so many different ways. Depending on which ones I have available and what flavors and textures I'm looking for, I use them when making breads, casseroles, omelettes, granola, juices, Asian dishes, pancakes, salads, sandwiches, snacks, soups, and tortillas. Experiment! See which sprouts you like best, and start including them in your recipes.

Happy Sprouting!

"Until he extends his circle of compassion to all living things, man will not himself find peace."

— ALBERT SCHWEITZER

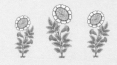

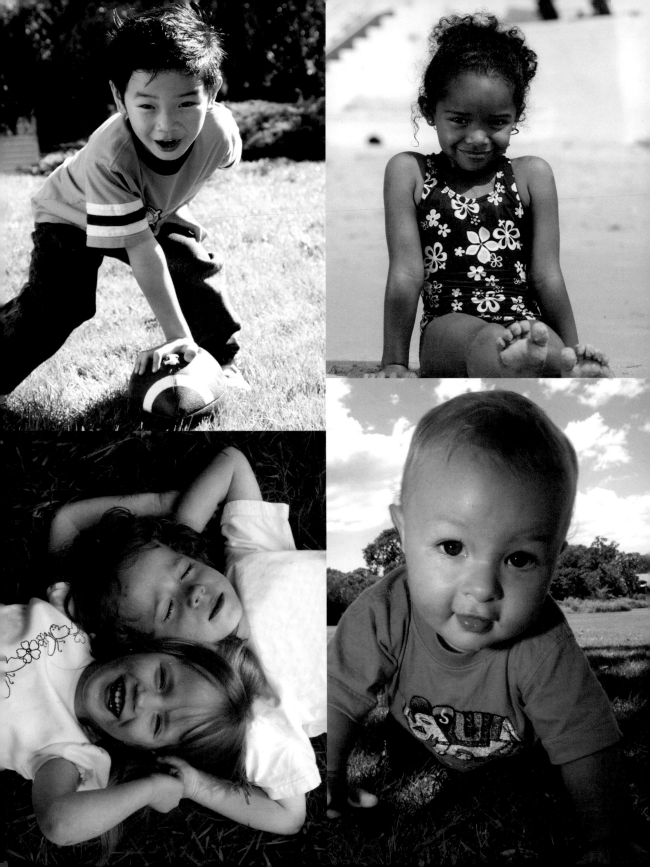

CHAPTER 13

RAISING CHILDREN TO BE VIBRANTLY HEALTHY:
12 SIMPLE TIPS THAT WORK

"We shall all be as good as dead one day, but in the interests of life we should postpone this moment as long as possible, and this we can only do by never allowing our picture of the world to become rigid."

— CARL JUNG

Hardening of attitudes is something that many adults succumb to. Yet the children in our lives teach us the importance of relinquishing our rigid outlooks and posturing. Being around young children is one of my favorite pastimes and enriches my life in so many ways; their approach to life is a gentle reminder to me that it's to be celebrated and enjoyed. But it's difficult for kids to enjoy themselves when they're unhealthy—as so many are these days.

When a child is born, a dream is born, too. What happens as the child grows up to fulfill that dream is dependent upon how the parent nurtures and nourishes. Ralph Waldo Emerson once wrote: "Health is our greatest wealth." That's certainly true for kids as well as teens and adults. While every child is different, I believe there are certain things that parents can do to expose their children to a healthier lifestyle.

Healthful foods and physical activity ride tandem as essential components to raising healthy children. Parents can easily suffer from information overload about food choices or become overwhelmed by their jobs, commuting, and stress-filled lifestyles. Although we as adults understand that good nutrition is important, many children actually eat a diet high in sugar and fat, low in calcium, and lacking in fresh fruits and vegetables. How our kids eat has a great deal to do with what they learn from the people around them. Similarly, they often duplicate the physical activity level of their parents. These messages are received in subtle and not-so-subtle ways.

A Balancing Act

Feeding children becomes a balancing act, and in many homes may turn into a battle zone. The more you force, the less they eat. Struggles create stress and conflict at the dinner table. But somehow we must get the message across to them about healthful eating and living.

A recent study from the University of Tennessee has shown that eating preferences are established by the age of three, so it's a matter of what you do with them early on. The younger your child is when you start this philosophy of healthful eating and living, the easier it will be later on. But whatever the age, it's better to start now than later. So what can parents do now to help make a positive, healthful difference in the lives of their children? Here are 12 tips that I've used for 25 years as a holistic lifestyle coach and health consultant.

1. Look at yourself first. It's essential for you as the parent or caretaker to make the necessary changes in *your* life since children learn best by example. You can't expect them to eat more fruits and vegetables if you never enjoy these foods or rarely extol their virtues. Be a shining example to your children.

2. Variety is the spice of life. Always have a variety of colorful fruits and veggies on hand, and let the kids help with the selection of produce in the market and the preparation of food at home. Studies show that the children who help create fresh meals are most apt to eat the dishes once they're prepared. This goes for school lunches, too. Let your child help you create a "power lunch" to take to school. Baby veggies and simple fruit, such as delicious satsuma tangerines or fresh berries, are easy to eat in a hurry (for a snack) and provide quick energy.

3. Take a fruit break. Every day, have your child take a fruit break. Fresh fruit—such as apples, oranges, berries, bananas, grapes, kiwi, tangerines, and pears—contains a plethora of nutrients, including enzymes, vitamins, minerals, antioxidants, and fiber. This high-water-content food is sorely missing in the diet of most children, who need at least three different fruits daily. If children take one such break during the day and add that to the fruit they'll have with breakfast and lunch, they'll be well on the way to enhancing their health and fortifying their bodies. In addition, take a daily veggie break together. Enjoy cut-up bell peppers, baby carrots, celery sticks, cherry tomatoes, string beans, or baby squash. Serve them with healthful dips. Strive for seven servings of vegetables. That's not hard to do when you have colorful salads and soups. Find ways to make these health breaks fun and rewarding.

4. Keep your home a junk-food-free zone. The saying "out of sight, out of mind" is certainly true when it comes to junk foods. Keep highly processed, refined products to the bare minimum at home. Let your child choose from a variety of fresh, whole foods rather than always deciding for them what they should be eating. In other words, give them back the power to choose, but make sure you offer them a variety of healthful options.

5. Break the food seduction. Processed foods—those high in sugar, white flour, salt, preservatives, and additives—are very addicting. The more they're eaten, the more they're craved. That goes for children, teens, and adults. It's best to begin each meal with a nutrient-dense, high-fiber food so that children receive nutrients before consuming any empty calories (items with high calories and little to no nutritional value).

6. Make quality sleep and plenty of water priorities. Lack of sleep and pure water exacerbates the craving for processed foods. Establish a nightly sleep routine, encourage ample water drinking, and offer a variety of whole foods. Feeling tired and cranky, lacking energy, or becoming moody is often a sign of dehydration and/or lack of sleep. Sleep, water, and the consumption of a variety of colorful, healthful foods need to be a nonnegotiable daily ritual.

7. Be prepared. Graze throughout the day on whole foods. This goes for children and adults. When the blood-sugar level drops too low, you'll crave anything that's quick and often devoid of nutrients. Keep plastic storage bags on hand, filled with healthful foods, so you and the kids don't become famished. Being very hungry distorts common sense.

8. Make the family dinner table sacred. Barring emergencies, have dinner together as a family, and don't use this time to discuss problems. Stressful meals impede digestion, suppress the immune system, and stifle joy and serenity. Mealtimes should nourish body and soul.

9. Join the breakfast club. Children need a healthful breakfast to start the day. *Breakfast* means "breaking the fast." If you feel rushed in the mornings, get organized the night before, perhaps by setting the breakfast table, making the lunches, laying out clothes, and organizing the morning meal. The first 40 minutes of each morning set the tone for the day. So fill your first 40 minutes with your family with organization, healthful foods, and fun.

10. Exercise as a family. Get involved with your children's favorite physical activities. Play basketball or soccer with them. Swim together, jog on the beach, hike the trails, or bike around the block. A family that exercises together stays healthy together.

11. Reward healthful choices. Find ways to reward your child when he or she makes choices to be more active physically—rewards such as extra quality time with you or with friends, a trip to the library or a movie, or a minute or two of TV time for every minute of exercise.

12. Encourage creative exercise. Invite your children to find ways to be more physically active—such as taking the stairs instead of the elevator, parking at the end of a parking lot when shopping, skipping together in the local park or beach before or after the family picnic, or exercising when watching television. If your children watch TV, do have them exercise at the same time. They can walk or march in place, or simply stand and stretch. I like to sit on the floor and stretch. It helps me stay flexible.

Pythagoras gave us this sage advice almost 2,500 years ago, and it's still applicable for children, teens, and adults alike: "Choose what is best; habit will soon render it agreeable and easy." Know that every healthful choice we make adds up. We are what we eat, how we exercise, and what we think. Happy children are healthy children, and vice versa. Choose to make health a top priority by being proactive. Let's love and protect our children and teach them how to live healthfully. They're our future, and they're worth it!

For information on my award-winning nutrition book for children, *Vegetable Soup/The Fruit Bowl,* co-authored with Dianne Warren, see "To Inspire & Empower" at the end of this book. To order *Farmers' Market,* a terrific board game for children that was created by Dianne Warren, visit: **www.fitness4kidz. com**. Both our book and Dianne's board game won the Disney iParenting Media Award for children's products.

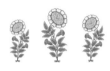

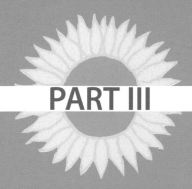

PART III

MAXIMIZE
YOUR HEALTH

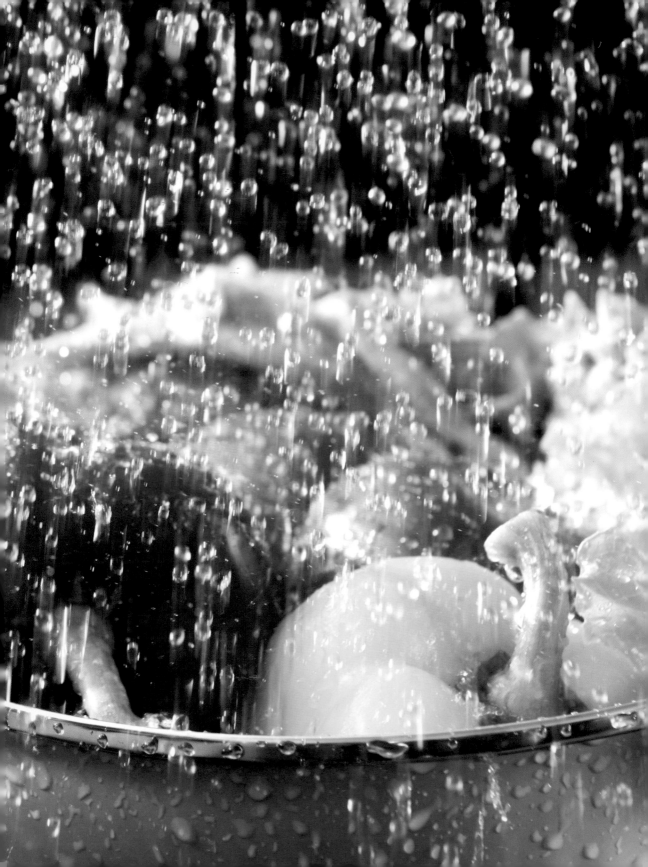

CHAPTER 14

VEGETABLE ENTRÉES

"He who distinguishes the true savor of his food can never be a glutton; he who does not cannot be otherwise."

— HENRY DAVID THOREAU

Vegetable meals are becoming more and more popular these days as the research pours in supporting the salutary effects of eating more plant-based foods as a way to heal the body and promote radiant health and youthful vitality.

The U.S. Department of Agriculture and the National Cancer Institute recommend a diet with at least 5 to 7 servings of fruits and vegetables every day to maintain good health. I suggest that you increase that amount to 7 to 12 servings daily. By incorporating the salads, smoothies, snacks, and soups from previous chapters, you're well on your way. Add the vegetable entrées you'll find in this chapter, and you'll be doing your body a big favor. In addition to the nutrient-rich vegetables in these recipes, you'll find other nutrient-rich foods, such as legumes, whole grains, nuts, and seeds.

Be Creative!

You can vary the ingredients in these vegetable entrées to create entirely new dishes. In fact, once you get the hang of it, you'll be making up your own recipes from scratch. With that in mind, don't be too concerned if you can't find one or more of the ingredients in a recipe; just substitute something similar. Cooking isn't exactly rocket science. You'll soon be very capable in your new, natural kitchen, as you already are in so many other areas of your life.

Now let's roll up our sleeves and get cooking!

SIMPLE & SUPER MARINARA SPAGHETTI SQUASH

This low-calorie, low-fat treat is easy to make and really delicious. Serves 2.

1 spaghetti squash, cut in half
1½ cups fat-free organic marinara sauce
½ cup mushrooms, sliced

Cover each half of the spaghetti squash with plastic wrap. In a microwave oven, cook until tender, about 12–15 minutes (about 40 minutes in a preheated 350° F oven). While the squash is cooking, add the sliced mushrooms to the marinara sauce and heat through. When the squash is done, scrape out the strands with a fork. (When scraped, spaghetti squash dislodges in strands much like spaghetti, hence the name.) Arrange them on a warmed plate and top with the sauce.

Variations: Substitute portabello or shiitake mushrooms for the regular mushrooms.

GRILLED OR OVEN-ROASTED VEGETABLE PACKETS

Combine your favorite vegetables in foil, place them on the grill or in the oven, and voilà: You have a scrumptious and very nutritious meal that only took minutes to prepare!
Serves 4–6.

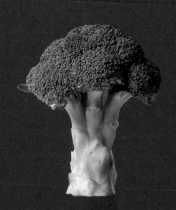

3 cups broccoli florets
1 cup cauliflower florets
1 medium onion, thinly sliced
1 yellow squash or zucchini, sliced diagonally
1 red bell pepper, sliced
1 tsp. dried basil
1 tsp. dried oregano
1 tsp. garlic powder
1 tsp. low-sodium tamari
1 tsp. cold-pressed, extra-virgin olive oil
3 ice cubes
1 sheet (18" x 24") heavy-duty aluminum foil

Preheat the oven to 450° F or the grill to medium-high. Place the vegetables on the center of the foil. Sprinkle with the seasonings and top with the ice cubes (to produce a steaming effect). Close up the foil by bringing the ends in to seal the packet, but leave room inside for the air to circulate. Bake on a baking sheet for 20–25 minutes or grill for 15–20 minutes. When serving, open the foil in front of your guests and wait for the compliments! Serve with a favorite grain such as millet, quinoa, or brown rice.

Variations: Substitute any combination of your favorite herbs for the oregano and basil, and add several whole cloves of garlic. Also, instead of drizzling the tamari and oil, combine these in a spray-pump bottle and spray lightly over the vegetables before cooking. This way you use less oil and distribute the oil and tamari more evenly. Try adding several diced red potatoes to the packet, and if you like hot and spicy, add some jalapeno peppers along with a dash of cayenne pepper and/or chili powder.

NORI VEGGIE BURRITOS

Nori are the sheets of seaweed used to wrap sushi. They make a delicious and mineral-rich "tortilla" that will hold just about anything you put into them. These little cross-cultural vegetable packets make a great portable meal. Nori sheets come either raw or toasted. I prefer raw, but if you like them toasted, you can do so yourself. Simply toast them in a large, dry skillet over medium heat for a few seconds on each side. They'll turn a light green color.

1 pack nori sheets (raw or toasted)
Sprouts of choice, such as alfalfa, red clover, sunflower, or mixed
Steamed vegetables of choice, such as carrot sticks, sliced mushrooms,
    or bell-pepper sticks
Sliced avocado
Tangerine-Ume Dressing (see Chapter 6) or your favorite dressing

Arrange a small amount of the vegetables, sprouts, and avocado slices on each sheet of nori. Top with the dressing. Roll up like a burrito or cone style. Seal the edge with a few drops of water. Eat whole or cut into strips. They may drip, so have napkins available. You can also wrap them with a napkin or foil and roll down the wrapper as you eat.

Sometimes I also add cucumber strips and sushi ginger (available in the Asian-foods aisle of your supermarket, Asian markets, and health-food stores).

FYI: Sea Vegetables

Sea vegetables such as nori increase the blood's alkalinity, which helps eliminate wastes and also may lower cholesterol, ward off certain cancers, control blood sugar in people with diabetes, prevent obesity and constipation, and fight hemorrhoids and diverticulitis. They're a potent source of iodine, a key factor in the control and prevention of many endocrine-deficiency conditions such as breast and uterine fibroids, tumors, prostate inflammation, adrenal exhaustion, and toxic liver and kidney states. Sea vegetables have no equals when it comes to major-mineral and trace-mineral content. Nori's subtle flavor makes it a great choice for those just beginning to experiment with these foods. You can purchase it in sheets that were dried naturally or already toasted, and in flakes that you can add to noodle dishes, soups, stir-fries, and salads.

ROASTED HERBED ASPARAGUS & POTATOES

There's nothing like the smell of roasting potatoes to make your kitchen feel warm and homey. Roasting the asparagus brings out a deep, nutty flavor.
Serves 3–4.

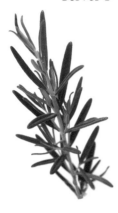

1 lb. small red potatoes
2 tsp. cold-pressed, extra-virgin olive oil
2 tsp. low-sodium tamari or Bragg Liquid Aminos
2 cups asparagus tops, sliced diagonally into 1-inch pieces
1 Tbsp. finely chopped fresh basil
1 Tbsp. finely chopped fresh rosemary
1 tsp. freshly ground red peppercorns
Freshly chopped basil for garnish
Nonstick cooking spray

Preheat oven to 400° F. In a large bowl or zip-top bag, combine the potatoes, oil, and tamari. Toss well so that the potatoes are evenly coated. Transfer to a shallow roasting pan that's been lightly sprayed with a nonstick cooking spray. Bake 40 minutes, stirring 3–4 times after the first 10 minutes of cooking. Add the asparagus, herbs, and pepper and bake an additional 15 minutes, or until the vegetables are tender. Sprinkle with the basil and serve with your favorite grain and/or beans and a crisp green-vegetable salad.

BROILED VEGETABLES

Almost any vegetable can be used in this recipe.
Serves 2–4.

1 cup zucchini, cut into ½-inch slices
1 cup eggplant, cut into ½-inch slices
1 cup mushrooms, cut into ½-inch slices
1 cup bell peppers, cut into ½-inch slices
1 Tbsp. Bragg Liquid Aminos or low-sodium tamari
Dash cayenne (optional)

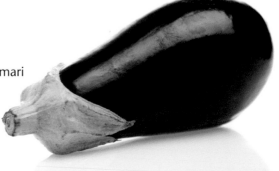

1 tsp. cold-pressed, extra-virgin olive oil (optional)
Nonstick cooking spray

Preheat the oven to 550° F and place the oven rack at its highest position. Combine the Bragg Liquid Aminos, cayenne, and oil, and brush lightly over the vegetables. Arrange the veggies on a baking sheet lightly sprayed with nonstick cooking spray and set on the top rack in the oven. Watch carefully so that they don't burn. Cooking time will range from 4–10 minutes, depending on the vegetables you're using. Thin ones (such as bell peppers, squash, or mushrooms) might brown faster, so lower the baking sheet one level. Check for tenderness, and don't overcook.

Variations: Add herbs such as dried rosemary, thyme, or basil to the vegetable mixture; or for some added zing, add minced garlic and/or minced ginger.

GINGER BROCCOLI & SHIITAKE STEAM-FRY

Using broth instead of oil to "steam fry," you cut the fat and calories in this vitality-promoting dish.
Serves 4.

1 orange, cut into pieces
3 Tbsp. Vegetable Broth (see Chapter 7)
1 Tbsp. low-sodium tamari or shoyu
2 tsp. minced garlic
2 tsp. minced ginger
1 small onion, minced
2½ cups broccoli florets, cut into 1½-inch pieces
1 cup shiitake mushrooms, cut into 1½-inch pieces
1 Tbsp. fresh orange zest (from an organic orange only)
3 Tbsp. fresh orange juice

Grate the zest off the orange, then cut off the rest of the peel and white pith and cut the orange into 1-inch pieces. In a large nonstick skillet or wok, heat the Vegetable Broth and tamari on medium high. (If you use shoyu instead of tamari, add it in the last 3 minutes of cooking only, not at the beginning, because extended heat diminishes its flavor and nutritional value.) Add the garlic, ginger,

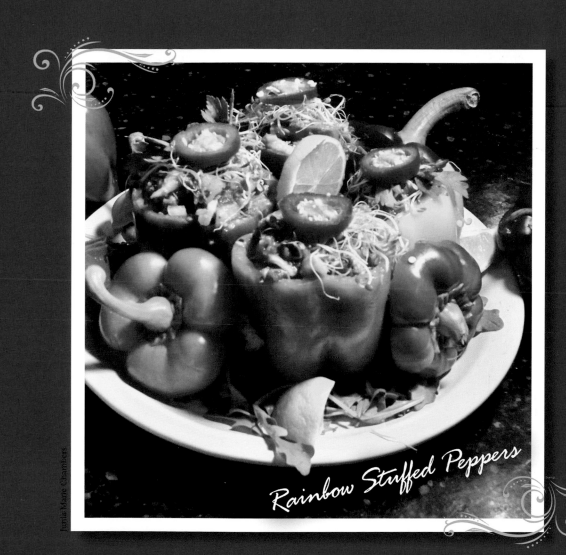

Rainbow Stuffed Peppers

and onion and cook for about 2 minutes, stirring occasionally. Add the broccoli, mushrooms, and orange zest and cook for 3 more minutes, stirring occasionally. When the broth has reduced by ¼, add the orange juice and orange pieces. Partially cover and simmer for 2–3 minutes, or until the broccoli is just crisp-tender.

FYI: Broccoli

Part of the cabbage family, like cauliflower, nutritious broccoli is prize worthy. It's slightly diuretic, contains twice the vitamin C of an orange, and almost as much calcium as whole milk—and its calcium is absorbed better. Broccoli contains selenium and vitamins A and E; and it's rich in chlorophyll, which is an excellent detoxifier and rejuvenator of the body. It's also considered the number one cancer-fighting vegetable. With almost no fat and just 12 calories per ½ cup (raw) and 23 calories (cooked), along with loads of fiber, it's a perfect diet food. Lightly steam a large batch to keep refrigerated to eat as a snack by itself, to dip, or to slice onto salads.

RAINBOW STUFFED PEPPERS

I love to make these peppers for company. The variety of colors is just a knockout.

Serves 4.

4 large sweet bell peppers in different colors
1 cup finely diced celery
3 ripe tomatoes, chopped
3 scallions, finely diced
1 large ripe avocado, mashed
1 carrot, grated
1 cup mixed sprouts
¼ cup diced jicama
¼ cup finely chopped green onions
1 Tbsp. Sesame-Seed Salt (also known as *Gomasio;* see Chapter 16)
Butter lettuce
Fresh parsley sprigs for garnish

Cut off the top of each pepper, remove the seeds and ribs, wash, and dry with a paper towel. In a bowl, combine all other ingredients. Spoon the filling into the peppers. Serve on a bed of lettuce or sprouts and garnish with fresh parsley sprigs.

Variations: When you're in the mood for something a little spicy, drizzle the stuffed peppers with a little salsa or add a chopped jalapeno pepper. Try using some fresh corn kernels cut off the cob or fresh peas. To add some extra protein, include some beans in the mixture or sprinkled on the lettuce leaves.

FYI: Bell Peppers

Sweet bell peppers are among the most nutrient-dense foods available. They supply impressive amounts of fiber and vitamins C and A, as well as silicon, an element that promotes beautiful hair, skin, nails, and teeth. With only 12 calories per ½ cup raw, they can be enjoyed raw, roasted, juiced, or added to a variety of recipes. They're definitely a superfood.

LETTUCE & VEGETABLE SANDWICH

While any lettuce will do, iceberg gives the most support.
Serves 2.

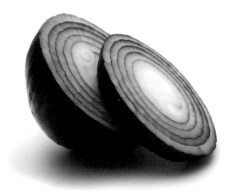

6 lettuce leaves, washed and separated
2 Tbsp. hummus
1 carrot, grated
1 medium ripe tomato, sliced
1 sweet onion, sliced
½ cup red clover or alfalfa sprouts
½ ripe avocado, sliced
8 cucumber slices
6 roasted cloves garlic, mashed (see Chapter 16)
8 roasted bell pepper slices (see Chapter 16)
Dash of sea salt

Remove the outer lettuce leaves carefully so you don't tear them. Use 2 pieces of lettuce for the bottom to give your sandwich more strength. Spread the hummus or other favorite spread on the bottom leaves. Distribute half of the remaining ingredients on top of the hummus. (Avocado helps hold the vegetables together.) Fold the leaves over the veggies, and wrap the third leaf over the top and around the bottom leaves. Repeat with the next sandwich. Use two hands and enjoy!

FYI: Lettuce

Lettuce is one of those excellent nutrient-dense foods that has virtually no fat and very few calories, but supplies your body with the necessary elements to keep it healthy and detoxified. Lettuce is alkalizing, cleansing, slightly diuretic, and contains the sedative lactucarium, which relaxes the nerves. It's a superlative source of magnesium, and along with bell peppers, contains the highest amount of silicon, which not only beautifies the skin, hair, nails, and teeth, but also supports pancreatic function. When you eat fresh fruits, I encourage you to also eat a fresh lettuce leaf such as romaine, which adds fiber, helps neutralize the sugar content in the fruit, and slows down the digestion.

CHOPPED BRUSSELS SPROUTS STIR-FRY

Here's a delicious and different way to serve one of the most popular vegetables—brussels sprouts.

Serves 4–6.

2 tsp. cold-pressed, extra-virgin olive oil
1 medium red onion, finely chopped
1 large carrot, finely chopped
2 cloves garlic, minced

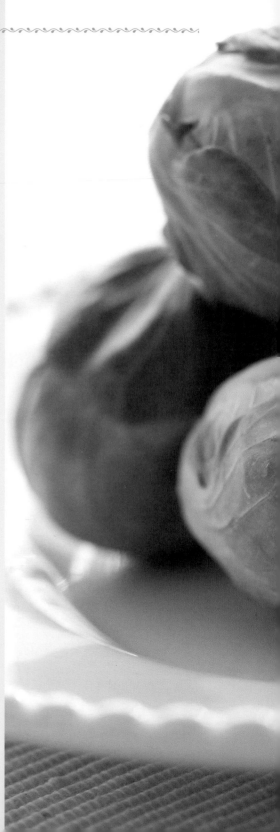

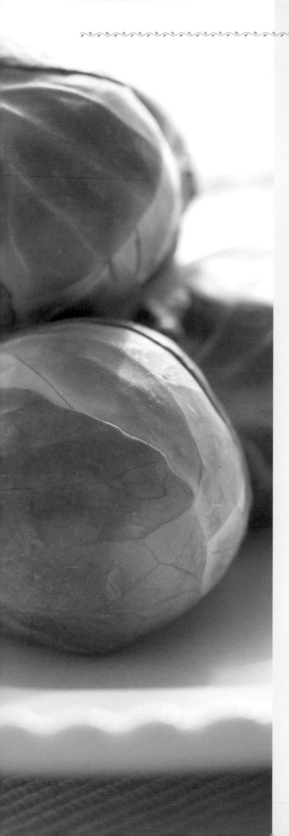

1 tsp. minced fresh ginger
2½ cups (1 lb.) chopped brussels sprouts
½ cup finely chopped jicama
1 sweet bell pepper (red, yellow, or
    orange), chopped
1 cup corn kernels, cut fresh off the cob
½ cup Vegetable Broth (see Chapter 7)
2 tsp. Dijon mustard
Sea salt to taste
Freshly ground pepper to taste.

In a large skillet, heat oil over medium heat. Sauté the onions until tender, about 3–4 minutes. Add the garlic, ginger, carrot, brussels sprouts, and jicama, and sauté for another minute, stirring often. Add the bell pepper, corn, and Vegetable Broth, and simmer for about 4–5 more minutes, or until the liquid evaporates, stirring often. Add the mustard, salt, and pepper, and cook for 1–2 more minutes. Serve on top of a bed of brown rice, quinoa, couscous, or millet alongside a fresh salad.

FYI: Brussels Sprouts

Brussels sprouts look like baby cabbages. Try them in stir-fries, soups, and baked dishes, or add them chilled (after steaming) to salads. You even can juice them. Like broccoli and cauliflower, brussels sprouts are at the pinnacle of phytochemical research, which shows them to be full of anticancer nutrients. They're rich in fiber, iron, protein, chlorophyll, calcium, and vitamins C and E, as well as being a superior source of vitamin U, an ulcer remedy. With only 30 calories per ½ cup, they're a nutrient-dense food that's perfect when fat loss and vitality are your goals.

ROASTED-VEGETABLE WRAPS WITH HUMMUS SPREAD

The combination of the roasted vegetables and the hummus spread makes this an equally easy and delicious meal for family gatherings, parties, or picnics.
Serves 6.

1 medium red bell pepper, cut into ¾-inch pieces
1 medium red onion, cut into ½-inch pieces
1 medium zucchini, cut in half lengthwise and
    then cut crosswise into ¼-inch slices
1½ cups mushrooms, cut into quarters
½ cup yellow squash, cut into ¼-inch slices
2 Tbsp. cold-pressed, extra-virgin olive oil
2 tsp. Bragg Liquid Aminos or low-sodium tamari
½ tsp. dried basil
½ tsp. dried oregano
½ cup hummus (see Chapter 4)
1 ripe avocado, diced
6 (8-inch) whole-wheat, fat-free tortillas, warmed
1½ cups shredded romaine lettuce

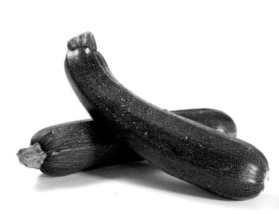

Preheat oven to 450° F. In a large bowl, toss together the vegetables, oil, Bragg Liquid Aminos, and herbs; then arrange in a shallow, nonstick roasting pan. Bake 12–15 minutes or until crisp-tender. While the vegetables are roasting, make up a batch of your favorite hummus and spread about 1 Tbsp. on each warmed tortilla. Place about ½ cup vegetable mixture in the center of each tortilla. Top with lettuce and diced avocado. Fold one end of each tortilla up about 1 inch over the filling. Fold sides in, overlapping over the folded end.

Variations: Use the same tortillas and instead of roasting vegetables, fill the wraps with all raw vegetables, such as lettuce, avocado, sprouts, tomatoes, cucumbers, onion, grated carrots, or any others you have on hand. I refer to this as my Rawsome Veggie Wrap. If you want to make it totally raw, replace the tortillas with a collard leaf or double-stacked (for strength) large leaves of romaine lettuce.

VEGETABLE, RICE & LENTIL CASSEROLE

Down home comfort food at its best.
Serves 4–6.

3 cups cooked short-grain brown rice
1¼ cups frozen corn
2 cups diced carrots
1 cup cooked red lentils
1 cup frozen peas
1 cup chopped green beans
⅓ cup chopped green onions
1 sweet red bell pepper, diced
2 cups Vegetable Broth (see Chapter 7)
2 Tbsp. Sesame-Seed Salt (also known as *Gomasio;* see Chapter 16)

Preheat oven to 350° F. In a bowl, thoroughly combine all of the vegetables and seasonings. Transfer to a covered loaf pan or casserole dish. Pour the broth over the mixture until it's just covered. Bake for about 20 minutes, or until it's heated through and the carrots are tender.

CHILLED ROASTED-VEGETABLE SALAD

Roasting the garlic, peppers, and onions brings out their rich nuttiness. They also give a wonderful visual and texture contrast to the crisp, fresh veggies in this summer salad.
Serves 4.

2 cups shredded romaine lettuce
1 cup grated daikon
1 cup shredded red cabbage
1 head garlic, roasted and squeezed out (see Chapter 16)
1 large onion, roasted and squeezed out (see Chapter 16)

4 sweet bell peppers, roasted and sliced into strips (see Chapter 16)
2 ripe tomatoes, cut into quarters
Vinaigrette dressing of your choice
2 Tbsp. toasted sesame seeds
1 lemon, cut into quarters

In a large bowl, combine the lettuce, daikon, and cabbage. Arrange on individual serving plates. Add garlic and onion, then crisscross the pepper slices over the top. Arrange the tomato wedges around the edges. Spoon on a small amount of dressing and sprinkle with toasted seeds. Garnish each plate with a lemon wedge.

RED CABBAGE WITH APPLES & PISTACHIOS

Over a bed of couscous or quinoa, this sweet and sour treat will wake up your taste buds.
Serves 4–6.

3 green apples, cored and sliced
1 medium-large head of red cabbage, sliced thinly (it's purple cabbage to me!)
1 onion, chopped
⅓ cup raisins
2 Tbsp. fresh lemon juice
1 Tbsp. brown-rice syrup
1 Tbsp. balsamic vinegar
¼ tsp. dried tarragon
¼ tsp. dried basil
¼ tsp. celery seeds
⅓ cup shelled, toasted, unsalted pistachios

In a large saucepan, combine all ingredients and cook for 25–30 minutes, covered, stirring from time to time. Serve with a salad of crisp greens and 3–4 vegetables.

VEGETABLE NOODLE DELIGHT

The soba noodles offer a delicious and healthful alternative to denatured white-flour pasta.

Serves 4.

2 large carrots, juiced
2 stalks celery, juiced
6 cups purified water
¼ cup Vegetable Broth (see Chapter 7)
1 medium onion, thinly sliced
1 large clove garlic, minced
1 large sweet bell pepper (red, yellow, or orange), chopped
1 tsp. dried basil
½ tsp. dried dill
⅛ tsp. sea salt
1 package firm or extra-firm organic silken tofu
2 Tbsp. yellow or light miso
Pinch of red chili powder
12 oz. soba noodles

Juice the carrots and celery and reserve ½ cup. (Drink any extra!) In a large saucepan or stockpot, bring the water and sea salt to a boil. In a large skillet, heat the broth over medium heat. Add the onion and sauté until tender, about 4 minutes. Add the garlic and sauté 1 more minute. Add the pepper and herbs, and sauté another 4 minutes—just until the peppers are tender. Meanwhile, in a blender or food processor, blend the carrot/celery juice, tofu, miso, and chili powder until smooth. Add to the sautéed vegetables and mix well. When the water comes to a boil, add the noodles and cook until al dente. (Check the directions on the package.) Drain, but don't rinse. When you rinse soba or pasta, you lose some of the flavor as well as the sticky coating that enables the sauce to cling to the noodles. Top with the colorful sauce and serve.

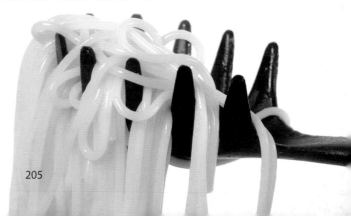

PACIFIC-RIM VEGETABLE STEW

As you savor this mixture of textures and flavors, you'll think you're across the world in a corner of paradise.
Serves 4–6.

1 small red onion, chopped
1 cup Vegetable Broth (see Chapter 7)
3 green onions, chopped
2 cloves garlic, minced
2 tsp. minced fresh ginger
3 ears of corn, kernels cut off the cob
2 carrots, sliced
1½ cups organic frozen edamame
1 lb. squash, such as yellow crookneck, sliced
1 large zucchini, sliced
½ lb. cherry tomatoes, cut in half
⅓ cup lite coconut milk
1 tsp. dried thyme
Shoyu to taste
Sea salt to taste
Cayenne to taste

In a large skillet over medium-high heat, steam-fry the onion with a dash of sea salt and ⅓ cup of the broth until the onions are tender, about 4 minutes. Add ginger, garlic, thyme, and green onions, and sauté another 1–2 minutes, stirring constantly. Add the rest of the vegetables, the remaining broth, and the coconut milk. Reduce the heat to medium, cover, and cook, stirring occasionally, for 12–15 minutes, until the squash and carrots are tender. A few minutes before the stew is done, add a teaspoon of shoyu along with a dash of cayenne to taste. Serve hot alongside couscous or jasmine or basmati rice.

STIR-FRIED HEARTS OF PALM & ARTICHOKE WITH SHIITAKE MUSHROOMS

This delicious, exotic combination can be pulled together anytime, especially if you keep a few cans of hearts of palm and a few packages of frozen artichoke hearts on hand.

Serves 4.

¼ cup dried shiitake mushrooms, rehydrated with hot water, drained, and sliced
2 tsp. cold-pressed, extra-virgin olive oil
2 cans organic hearts of palm, drained and rinsed, each heart cut into 3 pieces
1 package (8 oz.) frozen artichoke hearts, thawed, each heart cut in half
1 cup fresh pea pods
¼ cup Vegetable Broth (see Chapter 7)
1½ tsp. arrowroot or kuzu
1 Tbsp. low-sodium tamari
1 Tbsp. dry sherry
1 tsp. minced garlic
½ tsp. minced ginger

In a skillet over medium heat, stir-fry the hearts of palm, artichoke hearts, pea pods, and mushrooms in the oil for 1 minute. Add the broth, lower the heat, and simmer, covered, about 1 minute or until the vegetables are tender. In a bowl, combine the arrowroot/kuzu with the tamari, sherry, garlic, and ginger. Add to the vegetables and stir-fry until clear. Serve by itself or on top of a bed of couscous, quinoa, millet, or a combination of brown and wild rice.

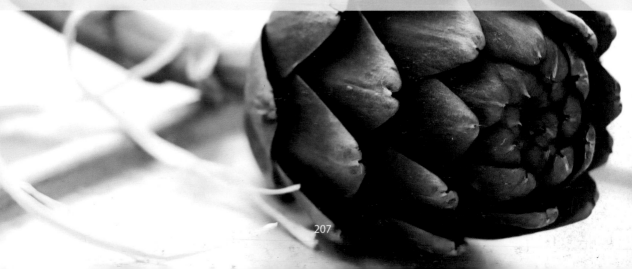

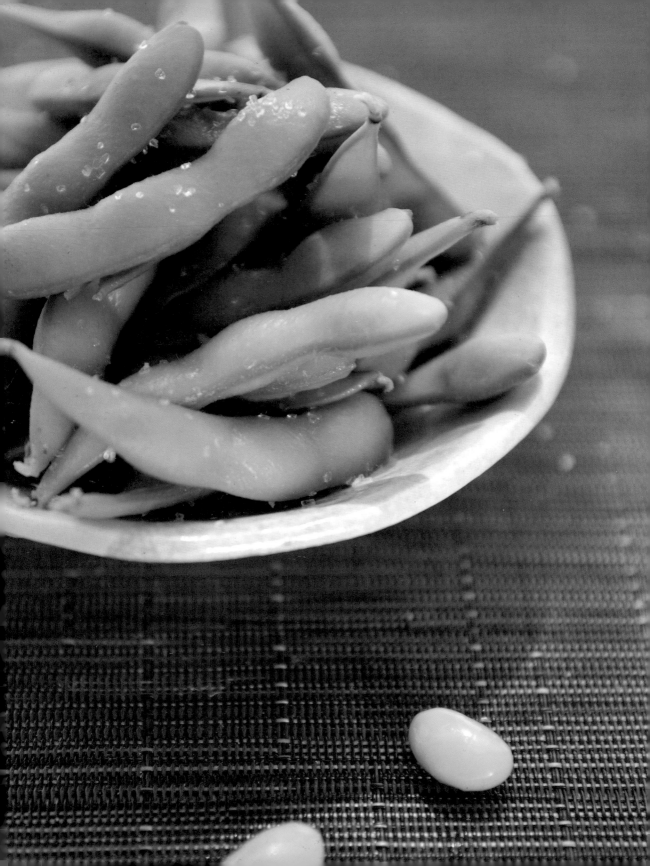

ROASTED CAULIFLOWER, EDAMAME & BELL PEPPERS

Roasting the vegetables brings out a wonderful sweet nuttiness.
Serves 4.

2 lbs. cauliflower
2 cups frozen shelled edamame (fresh soybeans), thawed, or lima beans
1 medium red bell pepper, cut into 1-inch strips
1 medium yellow bell pepper, cut into 1-inch strips
1 tsp. minced garlic
¼ cup Sesame-Seed Salt (also known as *Gomasio;* see Chapter 16)
Nonstick cooking spray

Preheat oven to 450° F. Place vegetables in a shallow, nonstick pan and sprinkle with the garlic. Spray lightly with a nonstick cooking spray. Bake 20–25 minutes, stirring a couple of times, or until you begin to see a tinge of brown. Place in a serving dish and sprinkle with Sesame-Seed Salt. Serve with a salad and a grain dish.

VEGETABLE-PITA PIZZA

These low-fat pizzas are fun for the whole family to make together.
Serves 4–8.

4 (8-inch) whole wheat pita breads, cut in half (around the edge)
2 heads of roasted garlic, squeezed out (see Chapter 16)
⅓ cup loosely packed fresh oregano
2 cups baby leaf spinach
24 cherry tomatoes, sliced in half
1 cup sliced mushrooms
1 yellow squash or zucchini, sliced
1 carrot, grated
1 package frozen artichoke hearts, thawed and chopped
1 sweet bell pepper, chopped
3 Tbsp. cold-pressed, extra-virgin olive oil
1 tsp. Bragg Liquid Aminos (optional)
1½ cups fat-free soy or other nondairy mozzarella, shredded

Preheat oven to 400° F. In a blender or food processor, purée the roasted garlic and oregano. Brush oil over the 8 pita shells. Arrange on a baking sheet and bake on the middle oven rack for about 5–6 minutes or until golden brown and crispy. Spread garlic-and-oregano mixture over the shells. Layer the shells with spinach, followed by the remaining vegetables. Cover with the cheese and bake 8–10 minutes or until all of the cheese is melted. For a saltier flavor, drizzle Bragg Liquid Aminos over the cheese after baking.

Variations: Some other great toppings are black beans (whole or mashed), sun-dried tomatoes, roasted onion and eggplant, imported sliced olives, roasted peppers, jalapenos, or lentils. In my book *Be Healthy~Stay Balanced,* you'll find recipes to make nondairy cheeses, such as a goat-like cheese, from nuts and seeds.

YUKON POTATOES, CORN & PEA ROAST

This roast is colorful, delicious, and so good for you!
Serves 4–6.

2 lbs. Yukon Gold (or Yellow Finn) potatoes, cut into 1¼-inch dice, unpeeled
1½ cups frozen peas
1½ cups frozen sweet corn
6 green onions, chopped
1 Tbsp. low-sodium tamari
2 tsp. cold-pressed, extra-virgin olive oil
2 tsp. organic balsamic vinegar
2–3 cloves garlic, minced
2 tsp. dried oregano
2 tsp. dried rosemary
1 tsp. minced ginger root

Preheat oven to 400° F. In a medium saucepan, parboil the potatoes for 5 minutes. Drain. In a small bowl, whisk together the tamari, balsamic vinegar, oil, garlic, ginger, and herbs. In a shallow, nonstick roasting pan, mix together potatoes, peas, corn, and green onions with the liquids. Roast for 15 minutes, or until the potatoes are tender, stirring a couple of times.

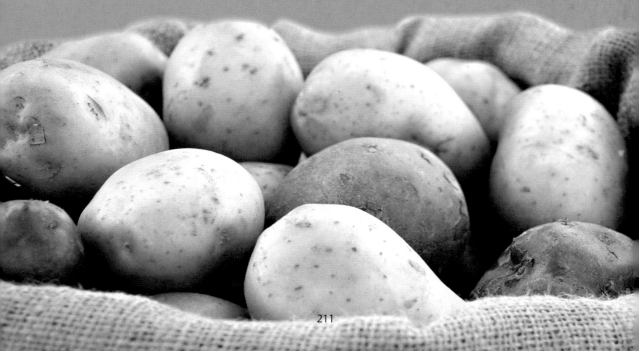

SOY-THAI-VEGETABLE SAUTÉ

If you like Thai food, you're in for a special treat. Serve this sauté over brown jasmine or basmati rice, a wild-rice mixture, couscous, or quinoa.

Serves 4.

1 medium onion, sliced
¼ cup Vegetable Broth (see Chapter 7)
1–2 tsp. minced garlic
Juice of 1 lemon
1 tsp. low-sodium tamari
2 red bell peppers, sliced
12 medium mushrooms, sliced
1½ cups thinly sliced broccoli stems
1 cup snap peas
½ cup sliced water chestnuts
1 cup (8 oz.) firm organic tofu, diced
1 (15-oz.) can baby corn
½ cup lite coconut milk
¼ cup soy nut, peanut, or almond butter
1 tsp. shoyu
2 tsp. minced fresh ginger root
Dash of cayenne and red chili flakes
Vegetable broth to thin (see Chapter 7)

In a large nonstick skillet or wok, combine the onion and the broth. Sauté for 4 minutes or until slightly tender. Add garlic, tamari, and lemon juice, and sauté 2 minutes longer. Add the remaining vegetables and tofu and sauté, stirring often, until crisp-tender. In a blender or food processor, purée the coconut milk, nut butter, shoyu, ginger, cayenne, and chili flakes. Use extra broth to adjust thickness. Pour over the vegetables, stir to coat, and heat through. Serve hot.

SHIITAKE MUSHROOMS, CARROTS & EGGPLANT SAUTÉ

I use shiitake mushrooms (fresh or dried) often for their scrumptious, earthy flavor.

Serves 6–8.

16 dry shiitake mushrooms, rehydrated in hot water and cut into strips
2 cups broccoli florets, cut into bite-size pieces
2 cups baby carrots, cut in half
2 cups eggplant, cut into bite-size pieces
12 oz. firm organic tofu, diced
2–3 large cloves garlic, sliced finely
2 tsp. fresh ginger root, minced
1 cup Vegetable Broth (see Chapter 7)
1 Tbsp. cold-pressed, extra-virgin olive oil
1½ Tbsp. shoyu or low-sodium tamari
1 Tbsp. chopped fresh thyme
1 Tbsp. chopped fresh basil
1 Tbsp. chopped fresh parsley
1 Tbsp. kuzu or arrowroot
3 Tbsp. purified water
½ cup toasted slivered almonds (or coarsely ground
    roasted cashews)

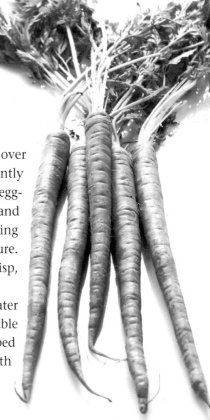

In a large nonstick skillet or wok, heat the oil over medium heat. Sauté the garlic and ginger, stirring constantly for 1 minute. Add the mushrooms, broccoli, carrots, eggplant, and tofu, along with ¼ cup of Vegetable Broth, and sauté for 5 minutes. Add enough water to the remaining broth to make 1¼ cups, and add to the vegetable mixture. Add the thyme, basil, and parsley. Cook until tender-crisp, about 5–6 more minutes.

Meanwhile, dissolve the kuzu in 3 tablespoons of water and add the shoyu/tamari. Add this sauce to the vegetable mixture and stir until the sauce thickens. Serve over a bed of brown and wild rice, couscous, or quinoa. Sprinkle with the toasted nuts.

RAW NUTTY-VEGETABLE PÂTÉ

With all of the walnuts, antioxidants, and scores of enzymes—because it's a raw-food recipe—you can consider this treat among one of your healthiest. I often serve it as a snack or appetizer with some pita chips; or for a festive entrée, you might stuff it into a hollowed-out tomato or bell pepper, or even a celery stalk.

Serves 8–10.

1 cup raw walnuts
1 cup raw pecans
1 cup raw sunflower seeds
1⅔ cups filtered water
1 Tbsp. yellow or sweet miso (optional)
½ cup shredded carrots
½ cup shredded zucchini
⅓ cup diced red or yellow peppers (or combination)
⅓ cup cilantro, chopped
⅓ cup parsley, chopped
2 tsp. chopped chives or scallions
Dash of cayenne pepper

In a food processor, purée the seeds, nuts, miso, and cayenne until creamy. Add the remaining ingredients and pulse gently to incorporate. If a thinner consistency is desired, add more liquid.

Tip: Vicki's Veggie Gobbler

If you are vegetarian or vegan, or just want to make a turkey-shaped pâté for the holidays, do what I do. I make it in a special turkey mold created by best-selling culinary author Vicki Chelf. To order, please visit: **www.vickisveggiegobbler.com.**

CHAPTER 15

GRAIN & BEAN ENTRÉES

"Let food be your medicine and medicine be your food.
Nature heals: the physician is only nature's assistant."

— HIPPOCRATES

Grains and beans are two of the best superfoods you can eat. Dried beans, peas, lentils, and chickpeas are collectively known as legumes. They have the most protein with the least fat of any known food, and they're high in potassium and low in sodium. A pot of beans, peas, or lentils is warm and filling; and when added to soups, stews, chilis, casseroles, or salads, beans and legumes strengthen the kidneys and adrenal glands and offer a great source of protein without adding cholesterol, saturated fat, or the toxic nitrogen byproducts found in meat protein. In fact, most legumes and beans contain 17 to 25 percent protein, higher than eggs and most meats. Soybeans rate exceptionally high in protein (38 percent), but soy products aren't ideal foods, so I keep them to a minimum.

Legumes are rich in potassium, calcium, iron, zinc, and several B vitamins, including folic acid, as well as the phytochemical diogenin, which appears to inhibit cancer cells. The soluble fiber in beans is very beneficial for reducing cholesterol, and their carbohydrates (because they're digested slowly and cause only a gradual rise in blood-sugar levels) makes them one of the best foods for people with diabetes or blood-sugar imbalances.

Whole grains are a top-quality energy food. They're complex carbohydrates rich in the B-complex group of vitamins: B_1, B_2, B_3, B_5, B_9 (folic acid), and biotin. Much is being written these days about avoiding grains and other complex carbohydrates if you want to lose weight. But there's a big difference between the unrefined carbohydrates in whole, natural foods and the refined carbohydrates in highly processed white flours and sugars. Whole foods haven't lost most or all of their fiber and other nutritional benefits like highly refined, low-nutrient products, such as white breads and pastas; sugary, fat-laden cakes; cookies; and other junk food have. For optimal health, eliminate white-flour products from your diet.

If losing weight is important to you, visit **www.4HealthBliss.com** to learn about and order a stellar weight-loss supplement that has been scientifically proven to help accelerate fat loss by lowering the level of the hormone leptin, making your body burn more fat. Also check out my Website, **www.Susan SmithJones.com**, and click on "Maximize Health" so that you can learn more about Max N•Fuze, MaxGXL, and MaxWLX and why most people would benefit from taking these three nutritional supplements.

The most nutrient-rich foods are dark, leafy greens. Nothing even remotely compares with them nutritionally. But they're low in calories, so we need to eat higher-calorie foods, too, to ensure that we don't get too skinny. Beans and legumes (along with fruit) are the next-highest nutritional categories, followed by grains, nuts, seeds, and avocados.

Add several servings of beans and whole grains weekly, and see how quickly your health and vitality blossoms.

SWEET LENTIL-PARSLEY SALAD

This salad makes a nice change from tabbouleh and is terrific by itself or spooned into warmed whole-wheat pita triangles.

Serves 5–6.

1½ cups dry lentils
¾ cup Vegetable Broth (see Chapter 7)
1 bay leaf
2-inch strip of kombu
1½ cups finely chopped, loosely packed, fresh Italian parsley

1 medium sweet onion, thinly sliced

2 sweet bell peppers (red, yellow, or orange), roasted, peeled, and cut into ½-inch strips (see Chapter 16)

2 tsp. lemon zest (from an organic lemon only)

¼ cup freshly squeezed lemon juice

⅓ cup minced fresh mint

¼ cup cold-pressed, extra-virgin olive oil or flaxseed oil

1 tsp. sea salt

¼ tsp. coarsely ground black pepper

¼ tsp. allspice

5–6 large purple or green cabbage leaves, for shells for the salad

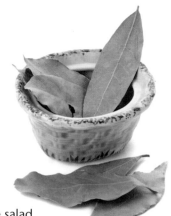

Rinse the lentils carefully and remove any small stones. In a large saucepan, combine the lentils, bay leaf, Vegetable Broth, kombu, and enough water to cover the lentils by 2½ inches. Bring to a boil. Reduce heat to medium low and cover. Simmer 20 minutes, just until the lentils are tender.

Place the onion slices in a colander and drain lentils over the onion to give it a natural softness. Discard the bay leaf and kombu, or you can cut the kombu into small pieces and add it to the salad. Transfer the lentils and onions to a bowl. Add the lemon zest and juice, parsley, roasted peppers, mint, oil, allspice, salt, and pepper to the lentils. Place a washed and dried cabbage leaf shell on each plate and heap several spoonfuls of the lentils on each leaf. Serve warm or chilled. Garnish with thin lemon wedges and warmed whole-wheat pita triangles.

FYI: Lentils

If you say you don't have time to properly cook beans, lentils are your answer. They don't need to be presoaked, take only minutes to cook, and have so little sulfur that they don't produce gas. Since biblical times, they've been a dietary staple; and their versatility makes them terrific in salads, soups, casseroles, stews, and side dishes. A cup of cooked lentils packs 16 grams of protein, whereas a 3-oz. patty of lean ground beef has only 15. And when you consider that lentils are very low in fat, whereas a burger has 18 grams or 162 calories of fat, you'll see why lentils are becoming more and more popular. They're also rich in iron, zinc, phosphorus, folic acid, calcium, potassium, and magnesium. This makes them a good source of nutrients for nearly every organ of the body, and they also aid in neutralizing acids. They help reduce blood cholesterol, control insulin and blood sugar, and lower blood pressure. There are many different colors to choose from, either whole or split and husked.

WHITE-BEAN & TOMATO CASSEROLE

Beans are very popular in Italian cooking. But whether you're Italian or not, everyone in your family will love this casserole.

Serves 6.

1 (28 oz.) can organic whole tomatoes, drained (reserve ½ cup liquid) and chopped
2 (15-oz.) cans of cooked white beans, drained and rinsed
1½ cups coarse, fresh, whole-grain breadcrumbs
2 red onions, finely chopped
2 large cloves garlic, minced
2 Tbsp. cold-pressed, extra-virgin olive oil
2 tsp. minced fresh parsley
1½ tsp. minced fresh tarragon
½ tsp. chili powder
¼ tsp. sea salt
¼ tsp. fresh lemon juice

In a small bowl, mix the breadcrumbs (chunks of dry whole-grain bread pulsed in a blender), 1 Tbsp. of the oil, the chili powder, dash of salt, and the lemon juice and set aside. In a large skillet, heat the remaining oil, add the onions, and sauté over medium heat until tender, about 3–4 minutes. Add garlic and sauté 1 more minute. Stir in tomatoes, tomato juice, beans, tarragon, parsley, and salt. Bring to a boil. Lower the heat and simmer for about 5 minutes, or until juice thickens.

Preheat broiler. Transfer the bean mixture to an 8-inch baking dish. Sprinkle breadcrumb mixture over the top of the beans. Broil for 3 minutes on the middle rack, or until the crumbs turn a golden brown. Be careful not to burn the top. Let it sit for 5 minutes, then serve.

Variations: Instead of tarragon and parsley, you can change the flavor by substituting other favorite fresh herbs such as basil, oregano, cilantro, chervil, cumin, or lemongrass; or you can give it a Tex-Mex twist by adding jalapeno pepper, chili powder, cayenne, and/or salsa.

GARLICKY QUINOA WITH CHESTNUTS & TOASTED PINE NUTS

Revered by the Incas as their mother grain, quinoa is an ideal high-energy, endurance, and fitness food that's easy to digest.

Serves 4–5.

2 cups water or Vegetable Broth (see Chapter 7) or a combination
1 Tbsp. lime juice
1 cup canned chestnuts, sliced and cut in half
½ medium red onion, chopped
3 cloves garlic, minced
1⅓ cups quinoa, washed 3 times and rinsed
    until the water is almost clear
1 Tbsp. minced fresh cilantro
3 Tbsp. pine nuts, toasted in a dry skillet
Sea salt to taste

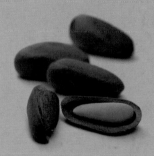

In a medium saucepan, steam-fry the chestnuts and onion with lime juice and 1 Tbsp. of the Vegetable Broth, until tender. Add the garlic and cook 1 more minute. Add the rest of the water or broth and bring to a boil. Add the washed quinoa and return to a boil. Cover. Lower the heat and simmer about 12 minutes. Add the cilantro, pine nuts, and salt to taste, then stir. Cover and remove from heat. Let stand 5 more minutes. Fluff with a fork and serve warm or chilled.

Tip: Chestnuts

Chestnuts roasted on an open fire, as the song implies, are as fun to eat as they are nutritionally beneficial. They're more like a grain or bean than a nut because of their high carbohydrate content and their low oil content, making them the most easily digested nut. Available fresh, dried, fresh-frozen, bottled, or canned, either whole or puréed, they add a nice crunchiness to any dish. You can boil them, roast them, mash them like potatoes, sweeten, or purée them. I like them sliced or diced in salads, dressings, and stir-fries, or grated and added to green beans, mushrooms, and peas. One of their virtues is that they stay crisp after cooking.

Chestnuts are sweet like a fruit, but unlike fruit, they build and warm, rather than cool and cleanse. They help strengthen tendons and nourish the stomach, spleen, liver, and pancreas. They have virtually no fat, so keep a few cans in your pantry.

COCONUT-RICE ALMONDINE

The coconut and almonds lend sophistication to this rice dish.
Serves 4.

¼ cup broth (see Chapter 7)
Dash low-sodium tamari or Bragg Liquid Aminos
1 cup chopped onion
2 cloves garlic, minced
2¼ cups water
1 cup lite coconut milk
1 Tbsp. fresh lemon juice
1½ cups short-grain brown rice
½ cup chopped mushrooms
3 green onions, chopped
⅓ cup chopped red bell pepper
3 Tbsp. slivered almonds, toasted in a dry skillet for 3–4 minutes
1 tsp. dried dill
½ tsp. dried parsley

In a saucepan, steam-fry the onion with broth and tamari for about 4 minutes. Add the garlic and cook for 1 more minute. Add the water, coconut milk, lemon juice, and rice and bring to a boil. Lower the heat and cover. Simmer about 35 minutes, until all of the liquid is absorbed. Add remaining ingredients; stir well; remove from the heat; and let stand, covered, for 5 more minutes. Fluff with a fork and serve.

FYI: Brown Rice

One cup of brown rice provides 5 grams of protein and only 230 calories. To get that much protein from steak, you'd need to consume a whopping 500 calories, which has lots of saturated fat as well. Calming to the nervous system and an impressive energy food, brown rice is rich in calcium; iron; magnesium; phosphorus; potassium; zinc; manganese; vitamins B_3, B_5, B_6; and folic acid. Keep in mind that brown rice is far superior to white because it retains its nutrition-laden, fiber-rich outer cover, which is better for stabilizing blood-sugar and insulin levels.

MILLET-TOFU SALAD WITH TOASTED PECANS

If you choose not to eat tofu or other soy products, you can still enjoy this recipe by using a nondairy, tofu-like firm "cheese." You'll find these products in a natural-food store, or you can make them yourself. Please refer to my book *Be Healthy~Stay Balanced* for a variety of nondairy recipes. I keep soy products to a minimum in my diet, eschew dairy, and make a panoply of foods that resemble dairy (such as yogurt, cheese, sour cream, milk, and cream), so I never miss dairy products.

Serves 4.

2 cups cooked millet
1 cup firm or extra-firm tofu, cubed and marinated
    in your favorite nonfat dressing

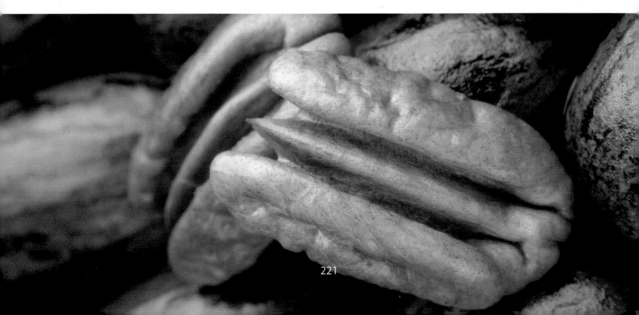

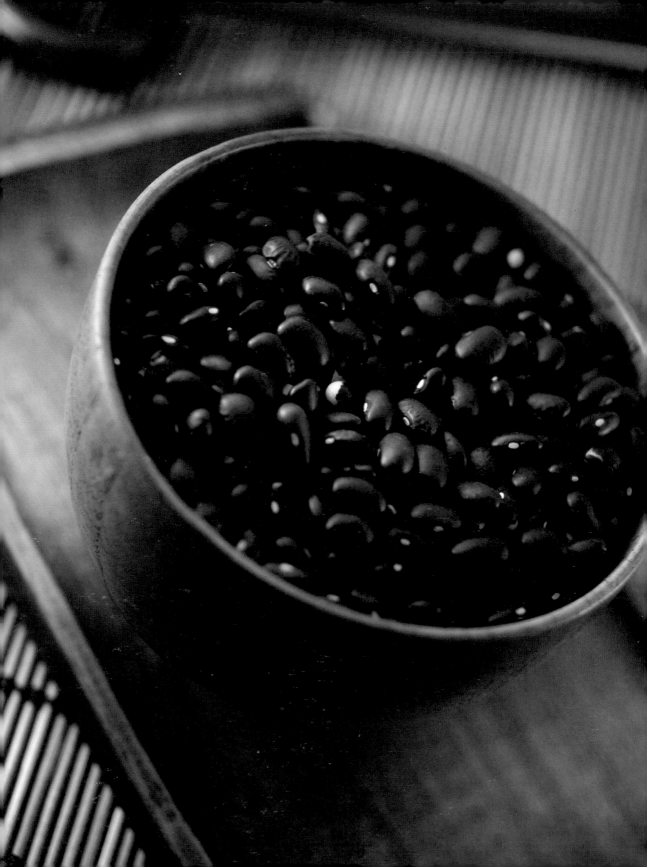

3 green onions, finely chopped
1 jalapeno pepper, roasted and minced
1 small clove garlic, minced
½ lime, juiced
½ lemon, juiced
2 Tbsp. chopped pecans, toasted in a dry skillet
2 tsp. finely chopped fresh cilantro
1 tsp. minced fresh ginger root

In a large bowl, toss all ingredients together and chill. Serve on a bed of crisp greens.

FYI: Millet

With only 50 calories in ½ cup, millet has the richest amino-acid protein profile and the highest iron content of all of the true-cereal grains. It's also very rich in phosphorus, magnesium, and potassium. Unlike wheat, it's gluten free; and due to its high alkaline-ash content, it's the easiest grain to digest and helps eliminate acidic wastes from the body. Great hot, warm, or chilled, this high-fiber, low-allergenic grain lends itself well to breakfast, lunch, dinner, or snacks. Toasting it for about 5 minutes, or until it begins to pop, brings out a nutty flavor.

ZESTY COUSCOUS WITH BLACK BEANS & CARROTS

Colorful and yummy, you can enjoy this dish as a snack, a side dish, or an entire meal.

Serves 3–4.

1¼ cups Vegetable Broth (see Chapter 7)
1 cup whole-grain couscous
1 (15-oz.) can black beans, drained and rinsed
1 cup carrots, finely diced
¼ cup minced fresh parsley
½ tsp. ground cumin
⅛ tsp. ground nutmeg

In a large saucepan, combine seasonings and broth. Bring to a boil, then remove from the heat. Stir in the couscous, followed by the beans and carrots. Let sit, covered, for about 10 minutes. Serve with salad that has lots of crisp greens.

FYI: Couscous

Couscous is a delectable, feather-light form of semolina wheat. Indigenous to North Africa, it's essentially a minuscule pasta that only takes 5–10 minutes to prepare. While not as nutritionally rich as other grains, it does provide fiber, some B vitamins, protein, and trace minerals such as zinc, iron, copper, and manganese. You can purchase it in bulk, but if you've never prepared it before, start with one package and follow the directions. Most packages contain too much sodium and seasonings for me, but it's a good way to learn how to make it. For best results, cook couscous in a wide pan. Both whole-grain and refined couscous are available, but I prefer the whole-grain variety for the extra fiber and nutrition.

BARLEY-LENTIL-CASHEW STEW

This is the perfect stew for cold winter nights—or anytime you want a hearty dish.

Serves 3–4.

1 cup Vegetable Broth (see Chapter 7)
1 cup water
¾ cup whole lentils
⅓ cup cashew pieces, toasted in a dry skillet
¼ cup barley
1 medium onion, chopped
6 large mushrooms, sliced
2 cloves garlic, minced
1 tsp. lemon zest (from an organic lemon only)
1 tsp. ground cumin
½ tsp. fresh lemon juice
Sea salt to taste

In a medium nonstick saucepan, sauté the onion in 3 Tbsp. broth. Add garlic and mushrooms and sauté 1 more minute. Add all of the remaining ingredients, stir well, cover, and simmer over low heat for about 50–60 minutes. Check periodically to see if extra boiling water is needed to make it the right consistency for stew.

FYI: Barley

Barley and wheat are the world's oldest cereal crops. Whole barley is a tan-colored grain, larger and plumper than all other grains except corn. While the bulk of barley is consumed in a malted form, otherwise known as beer, it's also a favorite in soup and stews. With only 200 calories per ½ cup, barley is a complex-carbohydrate energy food that has respectable levels of fiber and protein and low levels of fat. Whole barley is the most acidic of the grains, but can be made more alkaline and flavorful by roasting it a shade darker prior to cooking. Pearl barley has been polished, causing it to lose all bran and fiber and half of its protein, fat, and minerals. Purchase whole (unpolished) barley, and reap the benefits. Studies reveal that it lowers cholesterol and has powerful anticancer agents. It's also an excellent laxative.

ROASTED-GARLIC RISOTTO WITH SUN-DRIED TOMATOES & ARTICHOKE HEARTS

Risotto is elegant, rich, fragrant, and soothing. Most risotto recipes call for quite a bit of fat in the form of butter. This dish is low in fat without any sacrifice of flavor.

Serves 4–6.

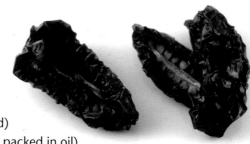

4 cups Vegetable Broth (see Chapter 7)
2 Tbsp. water
1 medium onion, minced
2 tsp. coconut oil
½ cup chopped artichoke hearts (frozen or canned)
½ cup chopped sun-dried tomatoes (not the ones packed in oil)
1 cup short-grain brown rice
1 head garlic, roasted, cloves squeezed out, and sliced in half (see Chapter 16)
½ cup dry sherry (or substitute sherry vinegar or nonalcoholic liquid)
3 Tbsp. fresh oregano, chopped
Sea salt to taste
Freshly ground pepper to taste

In a medium saucepan, bring the broth to a boil, then reduce the heat, cover the pan, and simmer gently. In separate saucepan, heat the oil and 2 Tbsp. water, then add the onion, artichoke hearts, and sun-dried tomatoes. Sauté until the onion is tender, about 3 minutes. Add the rice and garlic, then stir for 2 minutes. Add the sherry and cook, stirring constantly, until most of the sherry evaporates, about 2 minutes.

Add hot broth to the rice ½ cup at a time, stirring constantly, until most of the liquid is absorbed. Continue adding the broth until it's absorbed and the rice is al dente and creamy, about 20 minutes. Stir in the oregano, salt, and pepper. Serve hot.

BAKED JASMINE OR BASMATI RICE WITH CHICKPEAS

I usually double this recipe and freeze one casserole for a later date. Its buttery aroma and nutty flavor will make it a popular dish with family and friends. Of course, if you can't find jasmine or basmati rice at your natural-food store, brown rice will do just fine.

Serves 5–6.

2½ cups cooked jasmine or basmati rice
¾ cup cooked garbanzo beans (chickpeas)
1 small onion, chopped
⅓ cup sliced green onions
⅓ cup plus 2 Tbsp. Vegetable Broth (see Chapter 7)
2 cloves garlic, chopped
1½ Tbsp. nutritional yeast
1 tsp. coconut oil
1 Tbsp. low-sodium tamari
¼ tsp. paprika
⅛ tsp. ground cumin
¼ tsp. dried oregano

Preheat oven to 350° F. In a skillet, steam-fry the onion with 2 Tbsp. broth and a few drops of tamari for about 4 minutes. Add the garlic and cook for 1 minute. Transfer to a large bowl. Add the rest of the ingredients and transfer to a nonstick casserole dish. Bake uncovered for about 40 minutes. Serve with a salad.

GRAIN BURGERS

These freeze very well, so consider tripling the recipe so that you'll have lots on hand when you need them for burgers or to add to pasta sauces, on pizzas, or chopped into soups and stews.

Serves 6–8.

2 cups cooked millet
1 cup cooked short-grain brown rice
1 cup cooked quinoa
1 medium carrot, grated
2 cloves garlic, minced
½ cup grated zucchini
½ cup finely chopped red onion
¼ cup minced fresh parsley
1 Tbsp. Sesame-Seed Salt (also known as *Gomasio;* see Chapter 16)
2 tsp. unrefined coconut oil
¼ tsp. dried thyme
½ tsp. dried basil
⅛ tsp. ground cumin
Bragg Liquid Aminos or low-sodium tamari to taste

Preheat oven to 350° F. In a large bowl, mix all ingredients together using your hands. Form into 6–8 patties and place on a nonstick baking sheet. Bake for 15 minutes. Serve on whole-grain buns or on a bed of greens with all your favorite condiments.

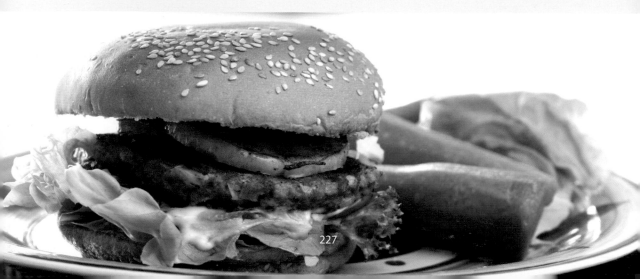

PORTABELLO-MUSHROOM CHILI

The wonderful, almost meaty flavor of portabellos stands up well to the strong spicing of chili. Serve this cozy stew on a cold night.

Serves 6–8.

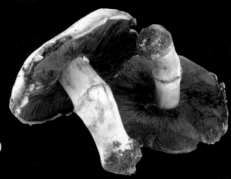

1 lb. pinto beans, soaked overnight, drained, and rinsed
3 cups water
3 cups Vegetable Broth (see Chapter 7)
4 small carrots, grated
3 large portabello mushrooms, finely chopped
1 (6-oz.) can organic tomato paste
1 large onion, finely diced
1 red pepper, seeded and diced
1 (2-inch) strip of kombu (remove before serving)
2 Tbsp. chili powder
2 tsp. ground cumin
1 bay leaf
1 tsp. sea salt
1 tsp. unrefined coconut oil or cold-pressed, extra-virgin olive oil
½ tsp. ground celery seeds
⅛ tsp. ground coriander
Cayenne pepper to taste (optional)

In a large pot, heat oil and sauté onion for 3 minutes. Add carrots and sauté 3 more minutes, stirring often. Add the remaining ingredients and cook, uncovered, over medium heat for about 10 more minutes. Keep stirring to prevent sticking. Add extra boiling water or Vegetable Broth if the chili gets too dry. This dish should be thick and rich.

Variations: Instead of portabello mushrooms, try ¼ pound of shiitake mushrooms, and if you like it really hot and spicy, add extra cayenne or chili powder.

> ## Tip: Portabello Mushrooms
>
> Portabello mushrooms are just a super-large version of cremini (aka "baby bello" or immature portabello) mushrooms you find in any supermarket. When they grow to this size, their flavor tends to intensify, becoming earthier and richer. They're fantastic grilled or sautéed and are a great substitute for beef or chicken in sandwiches, topped with lettuce, tomato, onion, and a couple slices of avocado, or a favorite spread such as hummus, Dijon, or Lemonaise (see Chapter 4).

MILLET WITH GARBANZO BEANS & VEGETABLES

The pale yellow millet is one of my favorite grains; and I enjoy it for breakfast, lunch, and dinner.

Serves 6.

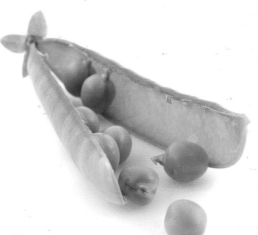

1 cup millet, rinsed and drained
2 cups water
½ cup Vegetable Broth (see Chapter 7)
1 small onion, diced
½ cup frozen corn, thawed
½ cup frozen peas, thawed
½ cup diced carrots
½ cup cooked garbanzo beans (chickpeas)
2 green onions, thinly sliced
½ tsp. sea salt

After rinsing and draining the millet, dry sauté it in a saucepan over medium heat, stirring constantly for about 4 minutes or until the millet starts to pop. Toasting will give it a nutty, full-bodied flavor. Add the water, broth, and salt to the millet, and bring to a boil. Lower the heat and simmer 10 minutes, covered. Add the corn, peas, onion, carrots, and garbanzo beans. Cover and simmer 10 minutes. Remove from heat, add the green onions, cover, and let sit for 1–2 minutes before serving.

Variations: Instead of garbanzo beans, substitute edamame, black beans, kidney beans, pinto beans, Northern beans, lima beans, sliced chestnuts, hearts of palm, or artichoke hearts.

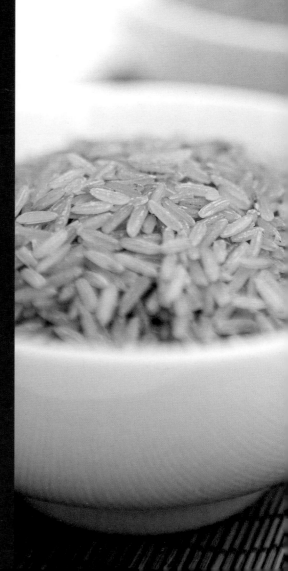

FYI: Millet

A study at the University of Minnesota suggested that middle-aged women who ate slightly more than one whole-grain food per day had a 15 percent lower death rate during the study than women eating lots of refined, processed grains. Millet is a whole grain rich in fiber and protein, easy to digest, and highly alkaline. This healthful "fast food" cooks in minutes.

SUSHI-RICE SALAD

Here's an easy way to incorporate nutrient-rich sea vegetables into your diet.

Serves 6.

1 cup Vegetable Broth (see Chapter 7)

2 cups water

1½ cups short-grain brown rice

2 medium carrots, diced

⅓ cup daikon, diced

4 nori sheets, toasted and torn into small pieces

¼ cup black sesame seeds

¼ cup cold-pressed sesame-seed oil

2 Tbsp. brown-rice vinegar

2 Tbsp. brown-rice syrup

1 tsp. Dijon mustard

¼ tsp. sea salt

Buy toasted nori sheets or toast them yourself. (See Nori Veggie Burritos in Chapter 14.) In a saucepan, bring broth and water to a boil. Add the rice and cover. Simmer over low heat 40–45 minutes, or until all of the liquid

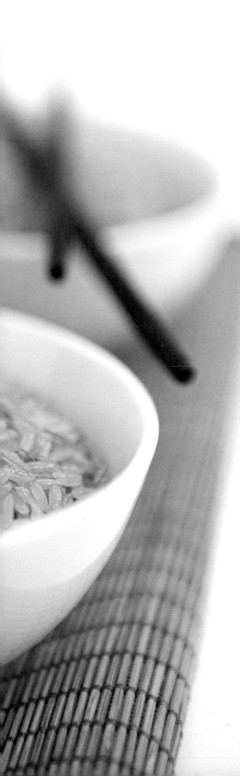

is absorbed. Uncover and let rice cool. Transfer the mixture to a large bowl and add daikon, carrots, and nori. In a small bowl, whisk together the sesame seeds, oil, vinegar, rice syrup, mustard, and salt. Pour over the rice. Serve on a bed of crisp greens.

Tip: Vegetable Broth

You'll notice that I often recommend vegetable broth as the liquid when cooking grains because it adds flavor and nutrients. You can find organic vegetable or mushroom broth in your health-food store or make it yourself in large batches and freeze it in plastic containers or zip-top bags. (See Vegetable Broth in Chapter 7.) Of course, if you don't have any broth on hand, you can always use water.

MARINATED BAKED TOFU SLICES

This high-protein recipe is great by itself or added to a variety of dishes. Try serving it with your favorite grain or to accompany a salad.

Serves 4.

1 lb. firm organic tofu
¼ cup shoyu or low-sodium tamari
¼ cup Vegetable Broth (see Chapter 7)
1 Tbsp. Dijon mustard
1 Tbsp. nutritional yeast
2 tsp. brown-rice syrup
1 tsp. minced garlic
Chili pepper to taste (optional)

QUINOA WITH LIMA BEANS, DRIED CHERRIES & TOASTED ALMONDS

You'll love the special flavor of dried cherries and toasted almonds in this resplendent recipe.

Serves 5–6.

1⅓ cups quinoa, washed 3 times, rinsed until the water runs almost clear, then toasted for 3 minutes
1⅛ cups Vegetable Broth (see Chapter 7)
1 cup water
½ cup cooked lima beans
⅓ cup chopped dried cherries
⅓ cup chopped almonds, toasted in a dry skillet
3 Tbsp. fresh orange juice
2 Tbsp. flaxseed oil
1 clove garlic, minced
1 tsp. lemon zest (from an organic lemon only)
1 Tbsp. fresh parsley, minced
1 Tbsp. fresh mint, minced
¼ tsp. sea salt

In a medium saucepan, bring the broth and water to a boil. Add the toasted quinoa and return to a boil. Lower the heat, cover the pan, and simmer about 12 minutes, or until all of the liquid is absorbed. Fluff with a fork, then stir in the beans, cherries, and almonds. Set aside for 5–6 minutes, uncovered.

While the quinoa is cooking, in a small bowl, whisk together the orange juice, oil, garlic, and zest. Then add half the parsley, half the mint, and the salt. Toss the dressing with the cooked quinoa. Transfer to a serving bowl or individual plates and top with the remaining parsley and mint. Serve warm, hot, or chilled.

Variations: Instead of lima beans, substitute soy, black, pinto, or kidney beans, or leave out the beans entirely. Try toasted sunflower seeds, hazelnuts, pumpkin seeds, or cashews. Instead of water or broth, use lite coconut milk or ½ almond milk (see Chapter 2), or use cold-pressed, unrefined coconut oil in place of the flaxseed oil to sweeten the dish a bit; you can also try extra-virgin olive oil or hemp oil.

Spicy Lemongrass Tabbouleh with Toasted Walnuts

FYI: Quinoa

Quinoa contains more calcium than milk and is high in the amino acid lysine, which may be scarce in a vegetarian diet. It's also a balanced source of other nutrients such as iron, phosphorus, B vitamins, and vitamin E and can be substituted in recipes for rice, millet, or couscous. It's great by itself as a side dish or as an ingredient in soups, casseroles, stews, pilafs, and even puddings. The flour can be used in breads, cookies, and other treats in place of wheat flour for those people with allergies. It also comes in a black color, which has a nuttier flavor than the lighter shades.

SPICY LEMONGRASS TABBOULEH WITH TOASTED WALNUTS

The Thai flavors in this salad lend an exotic twist to familiar tabbouleh. Serves 4–6.

2 cups boiling water
1½ cups bulgur (cracked wheat)
3 stalks lemongrass or 1 Tbsp. fresh lemon zest (from an organic lemon only)
1½ cups loosely packed, finely chopped, fresh parsley sprigs
½ cup loosely packed, finely chopped, fresh cilantro sprigs
½ cup loosely packed, finely chopped, fresh mint leaves
1–2 cloves garlic, minced
1 small red or sweet onion, finely chopped
1 large organic ripe tomato, chopped
⅓ cup coarsely ground walnuts, toasted in a dry skillet
¼ cup cold-pressed, extra-virgin olive oil
¼ cup fresh lemon juice
½ tsp. ground coriander
¼ tsp. cardamom
⅛ tsp. cayenne (optional)
½ tsp. sea salt
Mint sprigs for garnish

In a large bowl, combine the bulgur with 2 cups boiling water. Set aside for about 40–45 minutes, until all of the liquid is absorbed. Trim the lemongrass to

5-inch-long stalks, peel away outer layers, and coarsely chop the tender inside stalks. In a separate bowl, combine the lemongrass, parsley, cilantro, mint, and garlic. (I use a food processor with a knife blade to chop the herbs.) Add the chopped herbs to the bulgur (after all of the water is absorbed) and combine thoroughly. Add the remaining ingredients. Cover and refrigerate for 1 hour before serving. Garnish with mint sprigs and serve with warmed whole-wheat pita triangles, hummus, shredded carrots, and alfalfa or red-clover sprouts.

FYI: Walnuts

The most popular and widely used nut around the world, the walnut is rich in omega-3 fatty acids, which help reduce inflammation and alleviate pain. Being a nut, it's fatty (more than 60 percent) but it's still a healthful fat, mostly monosaturated and omega-3. It also provides protein, zinc, calcium, and potassium. Studies at Harvard University found that eating more than 5 oz. of nuts a week (not daily!) cut heart-attack deaths in women by 40 percent and helped prevent deadly irregular heartbeats in men. Walnuts also may help lower blood cholesterol. Like seeds, nuts are best eaten unsalted and raw. And if you want to lose lots of weight as quickly and healthfully as possible, limit your nuts and seeds to only 1 oz. daily, or 3–4 oz. spread throughout the week.

MEXICAN WILD RICE WITH OLIVES

The blacks, greens, reds, and yellows make this brightly colored salad a quick and beautiful dish worthy of guests.

Serves 2–3.

1 cup cooked wild rice
½ cup cooked brown rice
¼ cup diced sweet bell pepper (red, yellow, or orange)
1 large ripe tomato, diced
⅓ cup chopped fresh cilantro
¼ cup pitted and chopped black olives
2 tsp. cold-pressed, extra-virgin olive oil
1 tsp. chili powder
Juice of 1 small lemon
Sea salt to taste

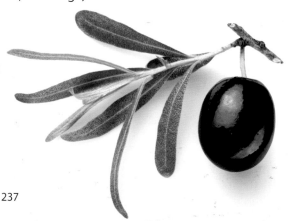

In a large bowl, combine all ingredients and refrigerate for one hour. Serve on a bed of lettuce. If you serve it with warmed whole-wheat pita halves, bring the dish to room temperature first.

Variation: I prefer to make this recipe with just the wild rice, and instead of cooking it, I sprout it and create a raw "living foods" nutritious meal that's wrapped in double butter-lettuce leaves and eaten with both hands. (See Chapter 12 for details on sprouting.)

FYI: Olives & Olive Oil

Olive oil is a major part of the Mediterranean diet. Researcher Ancel Keys declared olive oil the main dietary reason for remarkably low mortality rates among Mediterranean populations. Unlike other vegetable oils, it's high in antioxidant activity. For the freshest and healthiest, select organic cold-pressed, extra-virgin olive oil. It should smell sweet and light; a pungent odor may indicate that it's rancid. Always refrigerate oils to keep them fresh.

Olives acquired a bad reputation because of their high salt and fat content (up to 20 percent), but don't let that scare you away. You don't need to eat them by the handful, but a few added weekly to your favorite recipes is fine. They provide calcium, iron, and beta-carotene; are beneficial for the liver and gall bladder; and stimulate peristalsis.

Green olives are picked unripe, soaked in a lye solution, and cured in salt brine. In the past, the best olives came from the Mediterranean. Now, California produces excellent olives as well. Black olives mixed with your favorite spices make a great spread when puréed.

FYI: Wild Rice

Wild rice has a nutty, sweet flavor with a hint of spice. It's richer in protein, minerals, and B vitamins, and higher in carbohydrates than wheat, barley, rye, or oats. It's a warming food that's great for strengthening the kidneys.

LIMA-BEAN SAUTÉ

Even the pickiest eaters will ask for seconds of this recipe.
Serves 4.

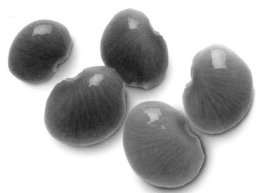

1 small onion, chopped
1 large ripe tomato, chopped
2 Tbsp. red-wine vinegar
1 Tbsp. cold-pressed, extra-virgin olive oil
2 tsp. low-sodium tamari
3 cloves garlic, minced
2 cups frozen lima beans
1 Tbsp. chopped fresh cilantro and parsley
    (combined to make 1 Tbsp.)

In a skillet, sauté the onion in vinegar, tamari, and oil for 3 minutes. Add the garlic and sauté 1 minute. Add the tomato and sauté 1 minute. Add the lima beans and sauté until heated through, about 3–4 minutes. Just before serving, toss in the chopped herbs and season to taste.

FYI: Lima Beans

As you probably guessed, lima beans gets their name from Lima, Peru, where they originated. Their flavor is similar to chestnuts, with a sweet and starchy taste; and they're used often in succotash, soups, casseroles, and as a side dish. I mash them like potatoes and use them in dips and spreads. They're beneficial for the liver and lungs, neutralize acidic conditions, and have less fat than most other beans.

CARDAMOM & PARSLEY BASMATI RICE

The rich color of this recipe makes it a feast for the eyes. The rich, lemony, aromatic flavor will get you breathing deeply and naturally, just to take in its essence.

Serves 4–6.

1½ cups basmati rice
6 cups water
⅓ cup chopped, loosely packed, fresh parsley
4–5 cardamom seeds
½ tsp. turmeric, ground
2-inch strip of kombu
2 bay leaves
1-inch cinnamon stick

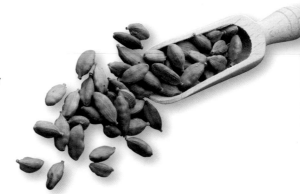

Wash the rice in a bowl of water and rinse until the water runs clear. Drain. Then soak the rice in 4 cups of water for 30–35 minutes. Drain. In a stockpot, combine the rice with 2 cups of water and all remaining ingredients. Bring to a boil. Cover tightly, reduce heat to very low, and gently simmer for 15 minutes, or until all of the water is absorbed. Turn off the heat and let the rice rest for 10 minutes, covered. Remove the kombu, cinnamon stick, and seeds. Serve as a side dish or with some beans and a salad.

Tip: Cardamom

Cardamom is a spice with a lemony zest and eucalyptus flavor that aids digestion. It's commonly used in Indian and Middle Eastern cuisines, especially in curries, desserts, and pilafs. I recommend purchasing cardamom in small green pods that have been air dried. Fresh seeds are plump and a uniform dark brown in color. Grind it yourself only in the amount needed because the flavor quickly becomes camphorous.

FYI: Turmeric

Also referred to as Indian saffron or yellow ginger, the rhizome, or root, of turmeric is bright orange, but otherwise it has the shape and skin of its relative, ginger. The highest known source of beta-carotene, it relieves inflammation, strengthens the immune system, and enhances digestion. An essential ingredient in curry, turmeric may be used to add color and flavor to any vegetable or grain dish. Buy in small amounts and store in a tightly covered dark-glass jar since light quickly reduces the color, flavor, and aroma.

GARBANZO, CARROT & TOMATO SALAD

I like to make a double batch of this recipe to have on hand when I feel like a quick yummy snack or to add to my salads or grains for a boost of protein, beta-carotene, folic acid, calcium, fiber, and omega-3s.
Serves 2–4.

2 (15-oz.) cans garbanzo beans (chickpeas), drained and rinsed
2 organic carrots, chopped
1 pint cherry tomatoes, sliced in half
½ medium sweet onion, chopped
1 Tbsp. finely chopped fresh parsley
2 tsp. flaxseed oil
2 tsp. organic balsamic vinegar
1 tsp. finely chopped fresh dill
Sea salt to taste

In a large bowl, combine all ingredients and refrigerate for one hour before serving.

SPICY SOUTHWESTERN BLACK-BEAN PATTIES

These "burgers" are great served with salsa on a bed of greens or with a whole-grain bun topped with salsa.
Serves 4–8.

2 (15-oz.) cans black beans, drained and rinsed
¼ cup organic cornmeal, extra if needed
2 Tbsp. unrefined coconut oil
¼ cup Vegetable Broth (see Chapter 7)
2 Tbsp. lime juice
1–2 cloves garlic, minced
1 small jalapeno pepper, seeds and white ribs removed, minced
2 tsp. chili powder
⅛ tsp. cayenne
1 tsp. low-sodium tamari

3 Tbsp. fresh cilantro, minced
1 Tbsp. Sesame-Seed Salt (also known as *Gomasio;* see Chapter 16)
1 Tbsp. cold-pressed, extra-virgin olive oil

In a large bowl, mash the black beans with a potato masher. In a small bowl, combine cornmeal, coconut oil, broth, garlic, jalapeno, chili, tamari, lime juice, cayenne, and cilantro. Add the liquid mixture to the mashed beans and purée. Stir in the Sesame-Seed Salt and add enough extra cornmeal so that you can shape it into 8 patties, each about 3 inches in diameter.

In a nonstick large skillet, heat the olive oil and cook the patties over medium heat until they turn a slightly darker shade, about 4–5 minutes on each side. You may want to add a little extra oil to cook the other side.

TOASTED HERB RICE WITH SHIITAKE MUSHROOMS

A heavenly aroma will waft through your kitchen as you prepare this enticing dish.

Serves 6.

3 cups short-grain brown rice
3¼ cups purified water
1¾ cups plus ¼ cup Vegetable Broth (see Chapter 7)
3 cups fresh shiitake mushrooms, sliced
   (or 1 cup dried, rehydrated in hot water)
1 tsp. dried dill
1 tsp. dried sage
1 tsp. dried marjoram
1 tsp. dried rosemary
½ cup sunflower seeds, toasted in a dry skillet
1–2 cloves garlic, minced (optional)
Bragg Liquid Aminos or low-sodium tamari to taste

In a large saucepan, bring the water and broth (except ¼ cup) to a boil. In a small bowl, combine the dill, sage, marjoram, and rosemary. In a large, heavy skillet, toast the rice and half of the herbs over medium-high heat, stirring constantly, until the rice is a shade darker, about 5 minutes. When the liquid comes

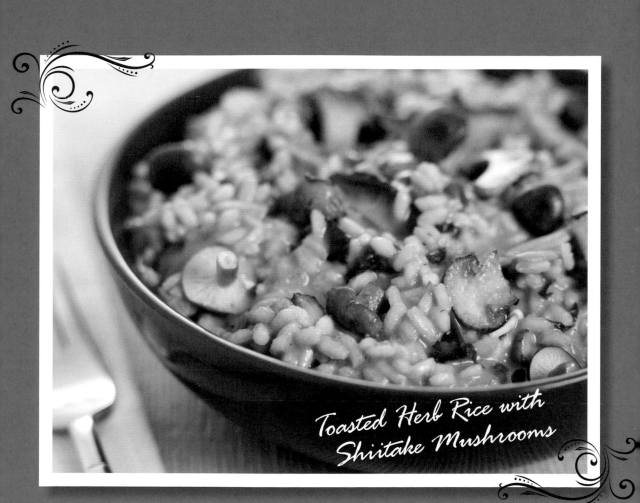

Toasted Herb Rice with
Shiitake Mushrooms

to a boil, add the toasted sunflower seeds and the toasted rice-and-herb mixture. Cover, lower the heat, and simmer until all of the liquid is absorbed, about 40 minutes. Remove from heat and let stand covered for 10 minutes. Steam-fry the mushrooms with the remaining herbs, the reserved ¼ cup broth, garlic, and Bragg Liquid Aminos (or tamari) for 7–10 minutes, or until the mushrooms are tender and heated through. Add to the cooked rice, stir, and serve immediately.

FYI: Shiitake Mushrooms

The second most widely produced edible mushroom, shiitakes have a rich woodsy flavor and meaty texture when cooked. Studies reveal that they contain substances that enhance the well-being of the whole body because they're rich in vitamins D, B_2, and B_{12} (rarely found in plant-based foods). You'll find them fresh and dried. To reconstitute, soak in warm water for 2–3 hours, preferably overnight. Use the soaking water for stock. Cut off the tough stem portion. Use shiitake mushrooms in stir-fries, entrées, side dishes, or pasta sauces, or grill them with marinade.

TOMATO COUSCOUS WITH CASHEWS & RAISINS

Serves 3–4.

2 cups fresh tomato juice (or organic, low-sodium bottled juice)
1 cup whole-wheat couscous
½ cup Vegetable Broth (see Chapter 7) or water
3 Tbsp. chopped sun-dried tomatoes (not the ones packed in oil)
1–2 cloves garlic, minced (optional)
⅓ cup raisins
⅓ cup chopped cashews, toasted in a dry skillet
2½ Tbsp. minced fresh parsley
¼ tsp. sea salt

In a saucepan, bring the tomato juice, broth, and salt to a boil. Add the rest of the ingredients, except for 1 Tbsp. parsley for garnish. Stir well. Cover, remove from the heat, and let stand 6–7 minutes. Fluff with a fork. Spoon into serving bowls or a platter, and garnish with reserved parsley.

CITRUS-BASMATI-RICE PILAF & MUSHROOMS

Citrus zest adds zing to recipes, especially this one.
Serves 5–6.

1 cup basmati brown rice
1 cup water
1 cup fresh orange juice
2 green onions, finely chopped
1 stalk celery, finely chopped
2 Tbsp. chopped favorite fresh herbs, such as dill, oregano, tarragon, chervil,
   thyme, marjoram, sage, parsley, or basil
2 tsp. unrefined coconut oil or cold-pressed sesame oil
1 cup shiitake (or button) mushrooms, sliced
2 tsp. fresh lemon juice
1 tsp. lemon zest (from an organic lemon only)
1 tsp. orange zest (from an organic orange only)
Sea salt to taste

In a large saucepan, combine rice, water, and orange juice and bring to a boil.
Then lower heat, cover, and simmer 40–45 minutes, until all liquid is absorbed.
Add all of the remaining ingredients and mix well. Let stand, uncovered, for 5
minutes. Fluff with a fork and serve.

Tip: Cooking Rice

The age of the rice determines how much water is needed to cook it. The older the
rice, the more water it will take. I use short-grain brown rice for stuffing, loaves, vegetarian sushi, and molds because it's stickier. I use long-grain brown rice when I want a
fluffier texture.

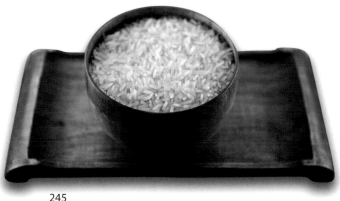

CHILLED MULTI-GRAIN SALAD WITH SWEET CORN

This salad mixes 4 grains and wonderful, sweet corn for a mouthful of interesting textures and flavors.

Serves 4–6.

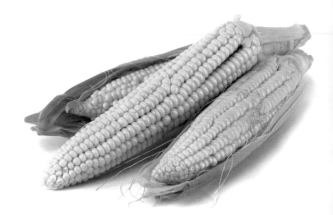

¾ cup cooked millet
¾ cup cooked short-grain brown rice
¾ cup cooked wild rice
¾ cup cooked quinoa
1½ cups frozen sweet corn, thawed
1 medium red bell pepper, finely diced
⅓ cup minced green onions (about 2)
¼ cup chopped black olives
¼ cup chopped fresh parsley
2 Tbsp. fresh lemon juice
2 Tbsp. flaxseed oil
Sea salt to taste
Freshly ground pepper to taste

In a large bowl, combine all ingredients. Refrigerate for at least 1 hour before serving. Arrange on a bed of greens and garnish with lemon wedges and sprigs of fresh parsley.

Variations: Instead of all of the grains combined, use a combination of just 1–2, such as brown and wild rice, quinoa and millet, or millet and couscous.

Tip: Buying Olives

Look for olives that are organic, cured in fresh water, and unrefined (still raw). Two of my favorites are Aragon black olives from Spain with a hint of thyme and Manzanilla olives that are cured for almost a year in fresh water, unrefined sea salt, thyme, fennel, garlic, and lemon. No vinegar, caustic acids, or dyes are used. Also available is Garum Organic Black Olive Paste from Spain, made from minced organic olives, olive oil, herbs, and unrefined sea salt. The paste is great on whole-grain bread or crackers, in salads, and on pasta dishes. (You can find the pastes in many natural-food stores.)

VEGETABLE-LENTIL-SWEET-POTATO CAKES

Serve these veggie cakes on a bed of lettuce greens or with a whole-grain bun. Serves 6–8.

3 cups water
2 cups Vegetable Broth (see Chapter 7)
2 cups yams, peeled and diced
1 cup dried lentils
½ cup uncooked short-grain brown rice
½ cup cornmeal
½ cup minced celery
⅓ cup grated carrots
⅓ cup diced zucchini
⅓ cup diced red or yellow bell pepper
⅛ tsp. ground cumin

In a large stockpot, combine all ingredients and bring to a boil. Lower the heat to medium and simmer 45 minutes, stirring occasionally, until lentils and rice are soft. Using your hands, form cooled mixture into 6–8 patties. In a nonstick pan, brown on each side, about 5 minutes each. You also can broil them.

ASIAN RICE

I love the Asian flavors in this easy rice dish. Serves 3–4.

1 cup water
¾ cup Vegetable Broth (see Chapter 7)
¾ cup brown basmati rice
1 (15-oz.) can French-cut green beans, drained and chopped
1 (8-oz.) can sliced water chestnuts
½ cup plain soy, almond, or hemp milk (see Chapter 2)
3-inch strip of kombu (remove before serving)
1½ Tbsp. Thai green-chili sauce
2 green onions, thinly sliced, for garnish
1 Tbsp. black sesame seeds, toasted in dry skillet, for garnish

In a medium saucepan, bring the water, broth, and kombu to a boil (remove kombu just before water boils). Stir in the rice, lower the heat, cover, and gently simmer for about 25 minutes, or until all of the liquid is absorbed. Meanwhile, in a skillet over medium-high heat, combine the green beans, water chestnuts, milk, and Thai sauce. Stir frequently while cooking, about 6–7 minutes. Serve over the hot rice. Sprinkle with the green onions and toasted sesame seeds.

FYI: Whole Grains

In a study conducted at the University of Minnesota, 36,000 healthy Iowa women aged 55–69 were given a questionnaire in 1986. After six years, 1,141 of the women were diagnosed with diabetes.

Those who consumed the most whole grains (average: 3 servings a day) had a 21 percent lower risk of diabetes than those who consumed the least (average: once a week). Those who consumed the most fiber (average: 10 grams a day) from whole-grain breads, cereals, and other grains had a 29 percent lower risk than those who consumed the least (average: 3 grams a day). For perspective, you should know that I get between 35 and 45 grams of fiber daily.

Finally, those who consumed the most magnesium, a mineral found in whole grains, had a 24 percent lower risk than those who consumed the least. So eat your whole grains regularly!

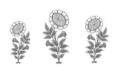

CHAPTER 16

SIDE DISHES & CONDIMENTS

"The wise man should consider that health
is the greatest of human blessings."

— HIPPOCRATES

This chapter includes some of my favorite small-portion recipes, which you can use in a wide variety of ways and settings. Whether you call them side dishes, appetizers, snacks, or treats is up to you. I've also included instructions on how to make some delightful condiments I refer to in other chapters. These can add savory flavors and rich textures to many meals. But be forewarned, they can only be used as condiments if you don't gobble them up the minute you make them. (They're that tasty!)

Whether your current dietary goal is fat loss or you just want to feel more energetic and look more youthful, it's best to stay away from huge meals, except for big green salads. As I explained previously, eating frequent, small meals throughout the day, as opposed to two or three large ones, revs metabolism, stabilizes blood sugar and mood, and helps prevent overeating.

Mixed Vegetables & Dips

For quick snacks whenever you need them, always keep a platter of mixed vegetables and a few favorite dips in your refrigerator. Along with fresh fruit, raw vegetables are the most healthful snacks you can eat. Don't limit yourself to celery, carrots, and cherry tomatoes. Reach out to green onions, bell pepper, cauliflower, broccoli, jicama, mushrooms, sweet onion, Belgian endive—anything that you can dip. Eat the vegetables raw, or lightly steam some (such as the broccoli and cauliflower) if you'll enjoy them more that way. But don't overcook them; make sure they're still crisp.

For the dips, see Chapter 4, or simply look for nonfat, low-sodium dressings at your natural-food store.

Now let's get started on the best little special-purpose recipes I know.

RAWSOME CRANBERRY RELISH

You can't get much healthier than this for a raw cranberry relish. I make it year-round to eat as a snack; on oatmeal, pancakes, waffles, toast, or muffins; or in my smoothies. By itself, it's divine, colorful, and zippy with its tart taste. It's one of my favorite snack foods because it's delicious and is so good for you. Every time I make it, it's a little different because I don't use exact measurements; I just eyeball it.

2 bags of fresh or frozen cranberries
1 medium pineapple, peeled, cored, and roughly chopped
One big handful raw walnuts
One handful of unsweetened, shredded coconut
Raw agave nectar (sweetener) to taste (I use very little)

In a food processor or blender, pulse until the berries are chopped and everything is mixed well. Place in a beautiful serving bowl for holiday meals or store in an airtight container in the refrigerator. It lasts for about 4–5 days, but it will probably be gone within a day or two.

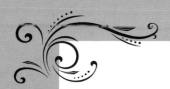

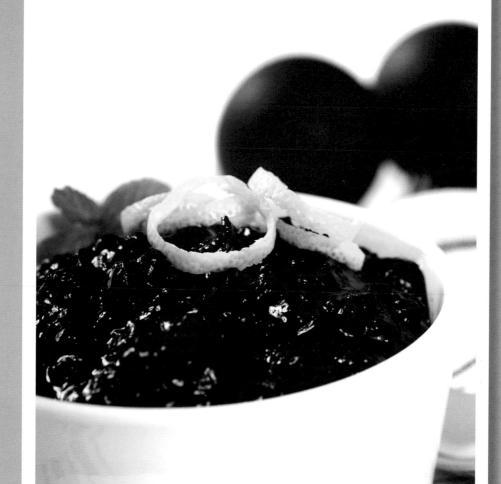

Rawsome Cranberry Relish

FYI: Agave

Extracted from the heart of the agave plant, agave is a low glycemic index (GI) sweetener, so it's slowly absorbed into the body, preventing spikes in blood sugar. It's 25 percent sweeter than sugar, so you need less. This sweetener has been consumed by ancient civilizations for more than 5,000 years. The mild taste is perfect for beverages, sauces, dips, smoothies, relishes, and baking. Agave is a terrific replacement wherever you use table sugar. It comes pasteurized and in unheated, raw forms. I always purchase the organic raw agave nectar at my local natural-food store; it's even available now in better supermarkets.

HERBED GARBANZO FLATBREAD

I use these for pizza shells, to accompany soup, or as a base for different spreads such as hummus and guacamole. Garbanzo flour can be found in most natural-food stores or made at home by grinding dried garbanzo beans in your food processor or The Kitchen Mill. (See the Resources section for ordering information.)

Makes 8 (5-inch) flatbreads.

1½ cups garbanzo flour
3 Tbsp. Sesame-Seed Salt (also known as *Gomasio;* see recipe in this chapter)
2 tsp. flaxseed meal
½ tsp. dried dill
½ tsp. dried rosemary
½ tsp. dried cilantro
Dash cayenne
⅓ cup Vegetable Broth (see Chapter 7)

In a bowl, thoroughly combine the garbanzo flour, Sesame-Seed Salt, flaxseed meal, herbs, and cayenne. Stir in just enough Vegetable Broth to form a dough ball. If you need extra liquid, use more broth or purified water, adding only a little at a time. Knead the dough for about 30–45 seconds, then divide it into 8 chunks and roll each into a ball. Place each ball, one at a time, between 2 pieces of plastic wrap and roll out from the center with a rolling pin or press out with your hands. In a nonstick skillet over medium heat, cook each one for about 2 minutes on each side, or until brown spots appear.

Variations: For a sweet dough, use water instead of broth and substitute 1 teaspoon cinnamon for the herbs. Top these flatbreads with applesauce or other fruit spread. For a heavier dough, use oat flour instead of garbanzo flour.

FYI: Garbanzo Beans

Garbanzo beans (chickpeas) have only one mature pea per pod and have a wrinkled, round surface. The high-protein flour is easily digested, and the whole beans have nearly double the amount of iron and more vitamin C than most other legumes (except soybeans, which do contain more iron). They're beneficial for the heart, spleen, pancreas, and stomach. In addition to including them in salads and making them into hummus, I also use them whole or mashed in soups, in vegetable and grain dishes, or just eaten plain. Simmer until tender, adding garlic and some toasted cumin seeds.

KALE CHIPS

Most people think of kale as a slow-cooked green that goes in soups and stews. Try this easy, fat-free, and wonderfully tasty way to eat kale and increase the calcium in your diet. Even kids love this special crunchy treat.

Serves 3–6.

10 kale leaves
Spice of your choice

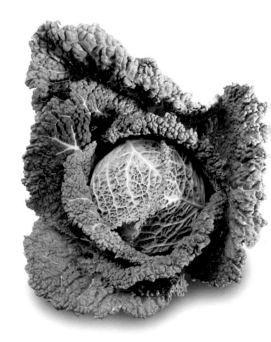

Preheat broiler. While the broiler is heating, wash the kale leaves, shake well, and pat dry with a paper towel. Lay them out on a broiling pan or baking sheet. Do not overlap them. Sprinkle leaves with your favorite spice or seasoning such as onion or garlic powder, cayenne, sea salt, ground cumin, or other herb-blend seasoning. Broil on a lower oven rack for 5–10 minutes, turning a couple of times. Kale burns easily, so watch them carefully. I use a spray-pump bottle and lightly mist the kale with low-sodium tamari before broiling. Serve warm or at room temperature.

> ## Tip: Kale
>
> Kale is a member of the cruciferous or cabbage family. The leaves are slightly curled and crimped (the word for kale in French translates as "curly cabbage") and strongly flavored. It can be juiced; steamed; sautéed; added to soups, stews, and stir-fries; or eaten raw in salads. It's an abundant source of calcium and chlorophyll and one of the best vitality and rejuvenating foods you can eat.

NO-OIL CHIPS & SALSA

An excellent alternative to regular, fat-laden chips.

1 dozen corn tortillas
Sensational Salsa or Festive Black Bean Dip (see Chapter 4)

Preheat oven to 375° F. Toast whole tortillas directly on an oven rack for 10–15 minutes or until crisp. Cut or break apart into quarters, and serve with salsa or other side dishes or dips.

ENTICING EDAMAME

Pronounced "ed-a-mah-may," this is one of the most popular snacks in Asia and a favorite appetizer in Japanese restaurants. These delicious young soybeans in the pod are a powerhouse of nutrients and just as fun to eat as they are simple to prepare.
Serves 3–6.

8–10 cups water
1 lb. frozen edamame
Seasoning to taste

In a large saucepan, bring water to a boil. Place the edamame in the boiling water and continue to boil. Cook 5 minutes over medium heat, uncovered. Drain. Lightly sprinkle with sea salt, spray with low-sodium tamari, or use any combination of your favorite seasonings. I like them plain.
Variation: Steam the edamame instead of boiling them.

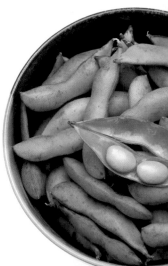

YUKON-GOLD POTATO SALAD

These special potatoes give this salad a delicious richness. There's no mayonnaise, so it's low in calories but high in fiber with lots of nutrients.

Serves 4–5.

2 lbs. Yukon Gold or new red potatoes (about 7 small potatoes) cut into 1-inch cubes, unpeeled
3 cups water
1¼ cups Vegetable Broth (see Chapter 7)
3 celery stalks, diced
1 sweet bell pepper (red, yellow, or orange), diced
⅓ cup diced green onions
¼ cup chopped fresh chives
¼ cup pitted and sliced black olives
¼ cup plain nondairy yogurt
¼ cup red-wine vinegar
1 Tbsp. chopped fresh dill
1 Tbsp. chopped fresh tarragon
⅛ tsp. sea salt (optional)

Place the potatoes in a stockpot and cover with the broth and water. Bring to a boil and cook until tender, about 20 minutes. Drain. Transfer the potatoes to a mixing bowl and set aside to cool. In another large bowl, combine the celery, bell peppers, green onions, chives, and olives. In a third bowl, blend nondairy yogurt, red-wine vinegar, dill, salt, and tarragon. Combine the potatoes, veggies, and dressing thoroughly. Refrigerate for 1 hour before serving. Arrange on a bed of crisp lettuce and garnish with fresh parsley.

Sweet & Spicy
Organic Baby Carrots

BROCCOLI COLESLAW WITH TOASTED SESAME SEEDS

This unique, colorful slaw is an antioxidant, anticancer, immune-boosting, delicious treat.
Serves 4–6.

3 cups broccoli stalks, lightly peeled and grated
½ carrot, grated
½ purple cabbage, grated
Favorite fat-free dressing
2 Tbsp. sesame seeds, toasted in a dry skillet

In a large bowl, combine everything except the sesame seeds. Divide the salad into individual serving bowls and sprinkle with the toasted sesame seeds.
Variations: Combine with red and yellow bell pepper, onions, and mushrooms. Sauté and wrap up in a whole-grain chapati (Indian flatbread) or tortilla.

SWEET & SPICY ORGANIC BABY CARROTS

The delicate flavor and texture of the baby carrots enhance this sweet dish.
Serves 4–6.

4 cups organic baby carrots
¼ cup agave nectar
¼ cup maple syrup
¼ tsp. cinnamon
¼ tsp. nutmeg
⅛ tsp. cayenne
1 tsp. chili powder
½ cup boiling water
Dash sea salt

Preheat oven to 350° F. Arrange the carrots in a casserole dish. In a small bowl, combine the syrups and spices. Add the boiling water and mix until blended. Pour over the carrots. Cover and bake for 1 hour.

FYI: Carrots

Rich in calcium, magnesium, potassium, and beta-carotene, carrots are a terrific detoxifier and an excellent food for the digestive tract, eyes, liver, kidneys, and immune system.

COLORFUL CUMIN-SPICED APPLE-CABBAGE WITH TOASTED WALNUTS

The distinctive taste of cumin adds the perfect flavor to this recipe. Serves 4.

1¼ cups plus 1 Tbsp. Vegetable Broth (see Chapter 7)
2 cloves garlic, minced
2 Tbsp. apple-cider vinegar
2 apples, peeled, cored, sliced into 8 pieces, then cut in half (16 chunks)
½ small head green cabbage, cored and sliced into ½ inch sections
½ small head purple cabbage, cored and sliced into ½ inch sections
2 Tbsp. chopped fresh parsley
1 Tbsp. low-sodium tamari or Bragg Liquid Aminos
1¼ tsp. ground cumin
1 tsp. chili powder
Dash cayenne
⅓ cup walnuts toasted in a dry skillet, for garnish

In a large pot, combine the Vegetable Broth, garlic, and vinegar, and bring to a boil over medium-high heat. Add the apples and cabbage and stir to combine. Cover, lower the heat, and simmer until tender, about 8–12 minutes, stirring occasionally. In a small bowl, combine the parsley, tamari, 1 Tbsp. broth, cumin, chili, and cayenne. Transfer cabbage mixture to a warmed serving bowl, toss with the spice mixture, and serve hot. Garnish with the toasted walnuts.

ROASTED-GARLIC & DILL-STUFFED MUSHROOMS

My friends rave about these stuffed mushrooms. They're easy to make, pretty to look at, and good for you. And who can resist the sweet and mellow taste of roasted garlic?

Serves 3–5.

15 large mushrooms, washed, stems removed
2 cups water
1 Tbsp. fresh lime juice
1 Tbsp. fresh lemon juice
1 tsp. lemon zest (from an organic lemon only)
¼ cup finely chopped red onion
1 Tbsp. plain soy or other nondairy yogurt
1 Tbsp. shoyu
1 Tbsp. Roasted Garlic (see recipe later in this chapter)
1½ tsp. dried dill
1 tsp. Dijon mustard

In a saucepan, combine the water with the lemon and lime juices, and bring to a boil. Add the mushroom caps and cook until tender, reducing heat to medium, about 10 minutes. Scoop out the caps with a slotted spoon and immediately plunge into a bowl of ice water to stop the cooking. Drain, pat dry, and arrange on a tray or platter. In a small bowl, combine the rest of the ingredients. Stuff the mushroom caps with the filling and refrigerate. Serve on a bed of whole Bibb (butter) lettuce leaves.

FYI: Dill

Dill has been used in herbal healing since the dawn of Egyptian civilization. In addition to its preservative action, it's an infection fighter and soothing digestive aid. The oil from the dill seeds inhibits the growth of bacteria that attack the intestinal tract and aids in relaxing the smooth muscles. It also helps alleviate intestinal gas.

FYI: Garlic

Garlic was recommended by Hippocrates for infections, wounds, cancer, leprosy, and digestive problems. Thousands of studies have been done on the salutary effects of garlic. As a natural antibiotic or nature's penicillin, nothing compares. And no standard medications even approach garlic when it comes to acting on so many cardiovascular risk factors at the same time. Some drugs reduce blood pressure, others decrease cholesterol, and some decrease likelihood of internal blood clots, which trigger heart attacks and some strokes. Garlic does all of these things, thanks to allicin and another chemical in the herb called ajoene.

STUFFED ENDIVE

Perfect to serve as an hors d'oeuvre to dinner guests.
Serves 4–8.

3–4 large Belgian endives
1 large carrot, grated
1 red bell pepper, diced
1 Maui or other sweet onion, diced
1 small rutabaga, diced
½ cup black olives, pitted
⅔ cup raw tahini
¼ cup fennel, diced
1–2 cloves garlic, minced
2 tsp. Dijon mustard
2 tsp. fresh lemon juice
Dash cayenne (optional)

Cut off the stems of the endive and separate the leaves. Rinse well and dry thoroughly. Arrange on a platter in a sunburst design. In a blender or food processor, combine the remaining ingredients and purée. Stuff the leaves and refrigerate before serving.

Variation: Try spreading some hummus on the leaves and top with a little salsa.

FENNEL-DILL SLAW

If you're tired of the same old coleslaw, this enzyme-rich variation will rekindle your interest.

Serves 4–6.

3 stalks celery, chopped
2 heads fennel, bottom core, tough parts, and leafy tops removed, finely sliced
1 small head purple cabbage, shredded
1 large carrot, diced
6 green onions, finely chopped
¼ cup fresh dill, finely chopped, or 1 Tbsp. dried dill
Lemon Tahini or Vitality Vinaigrette (see Chapter 6)

In a large bowl, combine all ingredients and serve with (or without) some of your favorite dressing.

FYI: Fennel

Fennel has been used medicinally for thousands of years. In the 3rd century B.C., Hippocrates recommended it to treat infant colic. Four hundred years later, Dioscorides called it an appetite suppressant. The Roman naturalist Pliny recommended fennel in 22 remedies, including one to help eye problems. These days, this aromatic herb is used as a digestive aid to help expel gas, treat diarrhea, and soothe the entire digestive tract (as an antispasmodic). It's also effective for women's health because of its mild estrogenic effect.

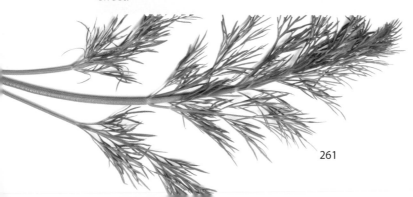

FANCY POTATO SKINS WITH SALSA

If you like Mexican flavors, you'll love these zesty double-baked potatoes.
Serves 4–8.

4 large baking potatoes, thoroughly scrubbed
1 small tomato, chopped
½ cup black beans, drained and rinsed
3 Tbsp. chopped green onions
2 Tbsp. Roasted Garlic (see recipe later in this chapter)
½ tsp. ground cumin
½ cup grated soy or other cheddar cheese
Sea salt
Freshly ground pepper

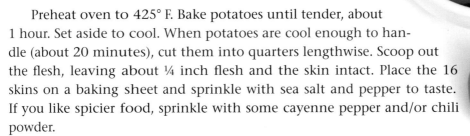

Preheat oven to 425° F. Bake potatoes until tender, about
1 hour. Set aside to cool. When potatoes are cool enough to handle (about 20 minutes), cut them into quarters lengthwise. Scoop out
the flesh, leaving about ¼ inch flesh and the skin intact. Place the 16
skins on a baking sheet and sprinkle with sea salt and pepper to taste.
If you like spicier food, sprinkle with some cayenne pepper and/or chili
powder.

In a small bowl, combine the tomato, beans, onions, roasted garlic, and
cumin. Spoon this mixture evenly on the skins, return to the oven, and bake
for about 3 minutes. Sprinkle with the cheese and bake until it melts, about 1–2
minutes. Don't overbake, or the potatoes will become dry and brittle. Serve with
some salsa, guacamole, and soy or other nondairy yogurt.

TOMATOES & ZUCCHINI WITH CILANTRO

This recipe makes a great topping for grains such as brown rice, millet, or
quinoa, or for potatoes.
Serves 4–6.

2 (15 oz.) cans diced tomatoes
1 lb. zucchini, sliced on the diagonal

2 Tbsp. Vegetable Broth (see Chapter 7)

2 tsp. cold-pressed, extra-virgin olive oil

2 cloves garlic, minced

¼ cup diced red onion

½ cup fresh cilantro, chopped

¼ cup chopped fresh spearmint or basil (or 1 Tbsp. dried)

In a large skillet, heat the oil and broth, and sauté the garlic, onion, and zucchini until translucent. Add the tomatoes and sauté until tender, 2–3 minutes. Add the cilantro and mint, and lower the heat and simmer, covered, for 3 minutes or until heated through.

Tip: Cilantro

Cilantro, the Spanish name for fresh coriander, looks like parsley but has a stronger flavor and is used widely in Mexican, Chinese, Thai, and Indian cooking. It's easy to find in most supermarkets, and remember: a little goes a long way. If the pungent flavor is too strong for you, you may substitute regular parsley for cilantro in any of these recipes.

STUFFED CUCUMBERS

This makes a refreshing appetizer, and a terrific snack or a delicious lunch served on a bed of greens.

Serves 3–6.

3 large cucumbers

1 cup minced celery

½ cup chopped orange bell pepper

½ cup chopped yellow bell pepper

¼ cup chopped green onions

½ cup raw tahini

2 Tbsp. minced fresh parsley (or cilantro)

1 Tbsp. fresh lemon juice

1 clove garlic, minced

Bragg Liquid Aminos to taste

Peel the cucumbers, then cut them in half lengthwise and remove the seeds with a spoon. Place the remaining ingredients, except the parsley, in a food processor or blender and blend everything together. Arrange the cucumber shells on a tray or platter. Stuff the cucumbers with the filling and refrigerate. Garnish with the parsley before serving. You can make the filling smooth or slightly chunky, depending on blender time. I prefer slightly chunky.

CREAMY-SPICY HERBED CORN

I like to serve this colorful corn dish with a grain such as quinoa or millet, along with a side of black beans, for a complete protein.
Serves 4.

3 cups fresh or frozen corn kernels
½ cup plain organic soy, almond, or hemp milk
3 Tbsp. Vegetable Broth (see Chapter 7)
⅓ cup diced red bell pepper
⅓ cup diced orange bell pepper
¼ cup diced red onion
1 jalapeno pepper, minced (remove seeds and white ribs if you don't
    want it super hot)
½ medium potato cut into chunks and juiced
1–2 cloves garlic, minced
1 tsp. ground cumin
½ tsp. dried tarragon
½ tsp. dried dill
¼ tsp. sea salt
Dash of cayenne pepper

In a large saucepan, combine the corn, milk, Vegetable Broth, bell peppers, onion, jalapeno pepper, garlic, and spices. Bring to a boil, stirring constantly. Cover, lower the heat, and simmer gently until the corn is tender, about 3–5 minutes, stirring occasionally. Add the potato juice and continue to cook over medium heat, until the sauce thickens, about 1–2 minutes.

CAULIFLOWER-BROCCOLI CURRY

Raw, crunchy, and satisfying, this curried snack is rich in antioxidants and vitamin C.

Serves 4–6.

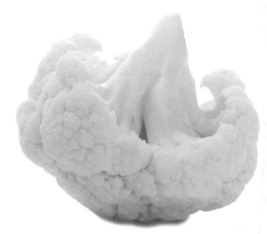

2 cups broccoli florets, cut into bite-size pieces
½ head cauliflower, cut into bite-size florets
⅓ cup cashew pieces
1 large Maui or other sweet onion, diced
¼ cup purified water
2 Tbsp. flaxseed oil
1 tsp. minced ginger
½ tsp. ground cumin
½ tsp. turmeric
½ tsp. shoyu

In a large bowl, combine the broccoli, cauliflower, onion, and cashews. In a small bowl, whisk together the water, oil, ginger, cumin, turmeric, and shoyu. Pour over the vegetables and toss to combine.

Tip: Fruits & Vegetables with Nut & Seed Butters

Simply spread your favorite fruits and vegetables with your favorite nut or seed butters for nutritious, quick, energy-boosting snacks. For fruits, select from apples, pears, bananas, or other favorites that lend themselves to being topped with a spread. For vegetables, celery is the best since you can spread the nut/seed butter into the center. Belgian endive, romaine lettuce, and quartered bell peppers work, too. If you have a juicer, you can make your own seed or nut butters. If not, you can buy them from the natural-food store. I prefer the raw varieties.

AUTUMN PURÉE

This colorful, antioxidant-rich, skin-beautifying snack or side dish is always a winner with everyone, from toddlers to seniors, and is fabulous served hot, warm, or cold.

Serves 3–4.

1 medium butternut squash
1 medium yam
3–4 medium carrots
Sea salt to taste

Cook vegetables (bake or steam) until tender and peel. They can be cooked with or without the skins—your choice. Cut into approximately 2-inch pieces. Purée the vegetables and season to taste. This healthful dish makes a perfect snack that lends itself well to lunch boxes or eating on the go. A few bites supply a treasure trove of nutrients. I usually double or triple the recipe and keep it on hand. It also makes a great spread for whole-grain toast and wraps, or a scrumptious dip for raw vegetables.

Variations: If you want it sweeter, use more yams. As you vary the vegetable amounts, you'll change the flavor slightly. Sprinkle on some cinnamon, nutmeg, or powdered ginger before serving, or garnish it with freshly chopped chives or mint and pecans, walnuts, or other nuts. For a special occasion such as Thanksgiving, add 1–3 Tbsp. pure maple syrup. (I use 1½ Tbsp.)

FYI: Yams and Sweet Potatoes

Although sweet potatoes are sometimes mistakenly called yams, the two aren't related. True yams are an entirely different kind of tuber. However, in the southern United states, a sweet potato is still called a yam. To further the confusion, canned sweet potatoes are also often misnamed. And although this food is labeled "potato," it's not in the same family as the common white potato! Whatever you choose to call them, they're both richly colored, naturally sweet, and highly nutritious.

ROASTED GARLIC

This simple-to-make treat is delicious and nutritious. A couple of times each week, you can smell garlic roasting in my home. Slowly baked, it becomes mild and so soft that you can spread it on bread like butter. Bake several heads at a time and keep them in the fridge, then warm them up in the microwave for a few seconds before using. I often squeeze all of the soft cloves from their skins and put them in a small bowl to use in a variety of dishes such as mashed potatoes, soups, salads, dips, spreads, sauces, and marinades.

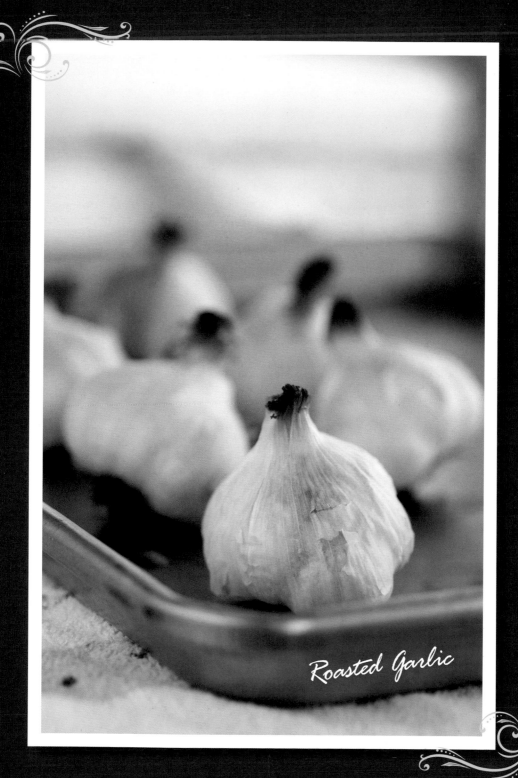

Roasted Garlic

6 heads garlic
½ tsp. dried thyme
½ tsp. sea salt
Nonstick cooking spray
Water

Preheat oven to 300° F. Slice ½ inch off the top of each garlic head (not the root end). Rub off as much loose garlic skin as possible without separating the cloves. Lightly spray a small baking dish with nonstick cooking spray. Place the skinned garlic heads, cut-side up, clustered together in the baking dish. Sprinkle the top of each head with a dash of salt and thyme. Add ¼–⅓ cup of purified water to the baking pan, surrounding the garlic. Cover and bake until the cloves are tender when pierced with a knife and beginning to pop out, about 1½ to 2 hours. Serve hot or cooled to room temperature.

I sometimes serve a whole head of garlic to each of my guests. They can squeeze out the soft cloves from the skins to spread on baguette toast or any variety of whole-grain breads, instead of using butter or margarine.

Variation 1: Instead of salt, drizzle some tamari or Bragg Liquid Aminos over the top of each head. It gives them a nice flavor and darker color. Or substitute other herbs such as oregano, rosemary, basil, dill, cilantro, chives, or cumin for the thyme.

Variation 2: Take 3–4 heads of garlic, separate all of the cloves, and peel away all of the skin. Discard any cloves that are very small. In a small saucepan, combine the garlic cloves with ½ cup Vegetable Broth (see Chapter 7). Bring to a high simmer, cover, reduce heat to a gentle simmer, and cook until the cloves are tender but not mushy, about 20 minutes. Check periodically to make sure the broth hasn't evaporated. If necessary, add some more. When cooked, the cloves are as soft as butter, easy to use, and will last 2–3 days in the refrigerator.

FYI: Garlic

Garlic is a superfood that has been studied worldwide for its medicinal properties. It's packed with antioxidants known to fend off cancer, heart disease, high blood pressure, and overall aging. It's also available in a supplemental form in a product called Kyolic. (See the Resources section for ordering information.) Kyolic isn't detectable on your breath, and I've been taking it since 1971. This is the best garlic supplement on the market.

ROASTED ONIONS

Like roasted garlic, roasted onions are easy to make and wonderfully delicious and versatile. Even kids love their mild taste. I roast several onions at a time to have on hand or to freeze. Enjoy them as a spread and as an ingredient in mashed potatoes, dips, soups, and sauces. You can use them whenever a recipe calls for onion.

Preheat oven to 400° F. Select onions of similar size (red, white, or yellow), and place whole and unpeeled on a baking sheet. Bake until tender and soft to the touch, usually about 25–30 minutes. Set aside to cool. With a sharp knife, cut off the root end and squeeze out the soft interior. Depending on the size, one medium onion yields about 1 to 1¼ cups diced roasted onion.

Variation: Place onion in a microwave on high or full power for about 5 minutes, or until soft to the touch. Set aside to cool. Cut off root end and squeeze out the soft interior.

FYI: Onions

With only 27 calories per ½ cup cooked, this flavorful, aromatic, and inexpensive food helps boost the beneficial HDL cholesterol, lower total blood cholesterol, retard blood clotting, and kill bacteria; it may even help counteract allergic reactions. When purchasing, make sure the onions are firm, dry, and well shaped. Avoid if soft or acrid-smelling. Store in a cool, dry place with good ventilation. I'm very fond of the sweeter onions, such as the Vidalia (Georgia), Maui (Hawaii), Sweet Texas, or Walla Walla (Washington) varieties.

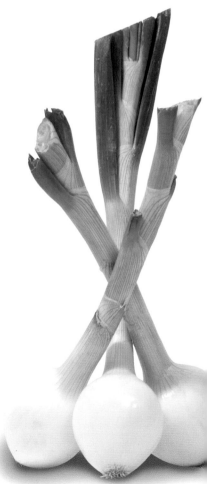

ROASTED PEPPERS

Roasting peppers is easy and brings out their natural sweetness. Select any color: red, yellow, orange, purple, or green.

Roasted peppers are easy to make. Simply place peppers directly on a gas stove-top burner, over a charcoal fire, or under a pre-heated broiler. Cook peppers on all sides, turning with tongs, until the skin blackens and blisters. Transfer the peppers to a heavy-duty plastic (zip-top) or paper bag, seal, and let sit for about 5 minutes. When cool enough to handle, peel away the charred pepper skin with your fingers. (Don't rinse the peppers under water because that will wash away some of the flavor.) Remove any discolored spots with a small sharp knife. Cut in half, remove seeds and ribs, and slice thinly.

Tip: Bell Peppers

The red bell pepper is the sweetest, but who can resist the luscious colors and refreshing taste of the yellow, orange, or purple ones? Because cooking makes the flesh of the purple peppers turn gray, it's best to eat them raw. The banana pepper is usually bright yellow, long, and tapered, but it can also be found in orange-red and green. Also called a Hungarian pepper, the banana pepper is great raw or cooked. I don't recommend eating raw green bell peppers, as they're merely unripe red peppers. Green peppers do roast well, however, so if you need a green color in a recipe, they might fill the bill.

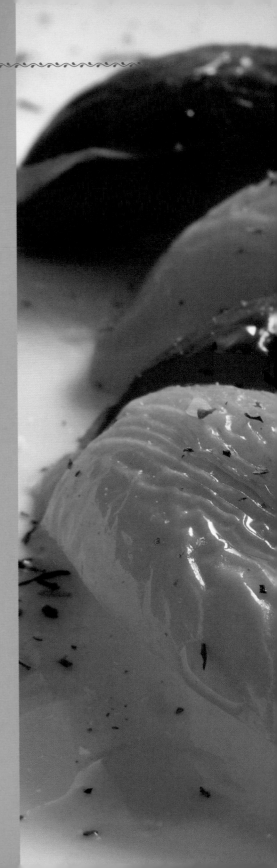

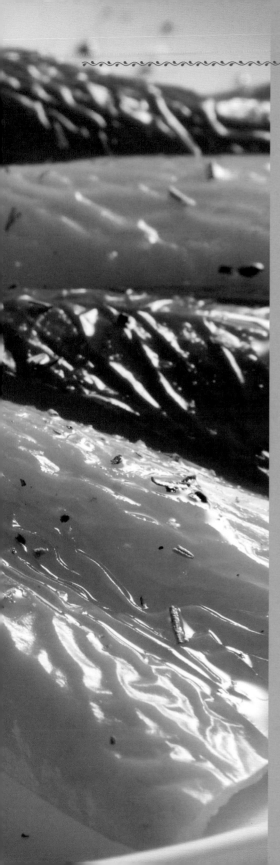

PLAIN CROUTONS

1 day-old baguette (preferably whole
    grain, nonfat), cut into ⅜-inch dice

Preheat over to 375° F. Arrange diced baguette on a baking sheet and bake for about 10 minutes, or until golden brown. Midway through baking, mix and toss the bread pieces. Cool.

Variations: Using a spray-pump bottle, lightly mist the diced bread with tamari before baking, or mist it with shoyu about 4 minutes before it's done. This will give your croutons a slightly salty flavor without too much sodium. I also dilute sea salt with a little purified water and mist the bread with this. To add color, juice any produce with the desired color you want and strain it carefully so you have only liquid; then mist onto the bread before baking. You also can spray an herbed olive oil from the spray-pump bottle.

HERBED CROUTONS

2 Tbsp. minced fresh parsley
2 tsp. minced fresh thyme
1 Tbsp. minced fresh basil
1 Tbsp. minced fresh chives
1 Tbsp. minced fresh oregano
1 tsp. paprika
1 tsp. onion powder
1 tsp. garlic powder
Dash cayenne pepper
⅓ cup Vegetable Broth (see Chapter 7)
2 Tbsp. cold-pressed, extra-virgin olive oil

1 Tbsp. Bragg Liquid Aminos or low-sodium tamari
12 slices day-old whole-grain bread

Preheat oven to 375° F. In a small bowl, mix together all of the herbs. In another small bowl, whisk together Bragg Liquid Aminos or tamari, oil, and broth. Combine the herbs with the liquid and mix well. Add enough extra broth to make the mixture brushable. Brush mixture on both sides of the bread. Cut into ⅜-inch dice and spread on the baking sheet. Bake until golden brown, about 10 minutes, tossing and mixing thoroughly halfway through the baking process.

Tip: Freezing Croutons

I make large batches monthly and freeze for later use on salads, in soups, as bread-crumbs, or as garnish in a variety of recipes. They thaw in minutes at room temperature.

FYI: Parsley

A relative of celery, parsley is the world's most popular herb. Because of its rich supply of chlorophyll, the green coloring in the plant, parsley is a superb blood purifier and overall body rejuvenator, which acts as a diuretic and even freshens breath when you eat a sprig of it. Parsley has three times as much vitamin C as oranges, and twice as much iron as spinach. It's also a good source of vitamin A, copper, and manganese. And because it's an alkaline food, it helps eliminate acidic wastes from the body.

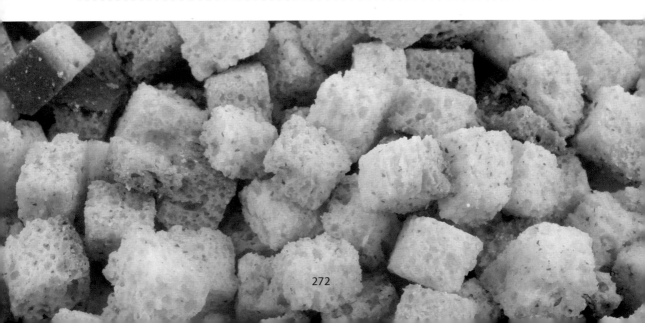

PEELED TOMATOES

Peeling tomatoes is a breeze to do and, in many recipes, yields a more elegant result.

Tomatoes
Bowl of ice-cold water

In a medium saucepan, bring purified water to a boil, making sure there's enough to completely cover a tomato. Immerse a tomato in boiling water for about 1 minute. With a slotted spoon, remove the tomato and immediately plunge it into a bowl of ice-cold water. Drain and peel the tomato. If the recipe calls for a peeled and seeded tomato, then cut the peeled tomato in half through the middle (the belly), and gently squeeze each half over a bowl to remove the seeds.

FYI: Tomatoes

Tomatoes are one of the very best sources of the antioxidant lycopene. According to studies, lycopene reduces the risk of cancer by 40 percent—notably prostate, lung, and stomach cancer—and increases cancer survival. In addition, research discloses that tomato eaters function better mentally in old age and suffer half as much heart disease. Concentrated tomato sauces (such as pasta sauces) have five times more lycopene than fresh tomatoes. Canned tomatoes have three times more than fresh!

ORGANIC GOMASIO (SESAME-SEED SALT)

Also referred to as sesame salt, I use this often because of the rich minerals it provides. It's delicious sprinkled on salads, noodles, soups, potatoes, grains, and cooked vegetables.

1 cup organic unhulled sesame seeds
1 tsp. sea salt

Wash the sesame seeds and drain well. In a dry skillet over medium heat, toast the sesame seeds for about 3–4 minutes, stirring constantly, until they start to pop. Reduce the heat and continue to stir and toast just until the seeds turn a shade darker, for another couple of minutes. Set aside to cool. Transfer the toasted seeds to a blender, add the salt, and grind in several on-off pulses until about 80 percent of the seeds are ground, being careful not to create a paste, which will happen if you grind even a few seconds too long! Transfer to a small, covered container. This stores well at room temperature for about 3–4 months. I use a tiny wooden spoon for serving and keep the spoon in the container.

Variation 1: To add more trace minerals and a different flavor, I make the recipe above and add ¼ oz. of dulse, wakame, or other sea vegetables. To try this, put the sea vegetables on a baking sheet and bake in a 350° F preheated oven for about 10 minutes, or until they start to brown. Cool. Blend alone until almost pulverized, about 12–15 seconds, then combine in the blender with the salt and sesame seeds.

Variation 2: Instead of sea vegetables, try variations of ground, toasted cumin, cardamom, cinnamon, fennel, fenugreek, mustard seeds, or black sesame seeds.

FYI: Sesame Seeds

Sesame seeds provide protein, calcium, iron, vitamins A, B_1, B_2, B_6, and niacin (B_3). Black sesame seeds have more flavor than white ones and are popular in Asian cooking as a garnish and also as an ingredient in many dishes.

GARAM MASALA

This aromatic spice mix is used often in Indian dishes and Ayurvedic medicine. It's known to help digestion and warm the body.

1 cinnamon stick (3 inches), broken into pieces
½ cup coriander seeds
1 cup cumin seeds
¼ cup fennel seeds
1 Tbsp. unhulled sesame seeds
2 Tbsp. black peppercorns
2 Tbsp. black cardamom seeds
2 Tbsp. whole cloves
2 tsp. sea salt

In a large, heavy skillet over low heat, toast all of the seeds and spices (except the sea salt), stirring often, for about 12–15 minutes, or until their aroma is released. Set aside to cool. (Your kitchen and home will smell heavenly!) Transfer to a spice mill or blender. Add the salt and grind into a fine powder. Sift through a fine sieve. Store in an airtight container in a cool, dry place for up to four or five months.

FYI: Cumin

As mentioned previously, cumin is a member of the parsley family. It has a pungent flavor that loses its essence quickly to become bitter tasting in most store-bought brands. Look for the whole cumin seeds and take the time to grind them fresh. Cumin is beneficial for the digestive system, improves liver function, promotes the assimilation of other foods, and helps relieve headaches and abdominal distention due to gas.

FYI: Pepper and Peppercorns

It's always best to grind peppercorns fresh; the taste is better and it prevents rancidity. Once ground, add pepper at the end of cooking to prevent the pungent flavor from becoming bitter. Pepper is a good source of chromium and acts as an anti-inflammatory and parasite inhibitor. In fact, when I have a cut or wound, I often sprinkle fresh pepper on it to reduce pain and swelling and to help it heal faster.

Black pepper is produced from the still-green unripe berries of the pepper plant. The green berry is cooked briefly in hot water to clean and prepare it for drying. Whether sun- or machine-dried, the fruit around the seed of the berry shrinks and darkens into a thin, wrinkled black layer, which is called a peppercorn once it's dried. The flavor is hot with a hint of spice and sweetness.

Green peppercorns are picked when mature but still green, and are packed in brine or dried. Red peppercorns have rose hips added for a color change and different taste. They're sweet and only mildly pungent. Because much of pepper's pungency is in its skin, which is removed when soaked in brine, white pepper's fragrance excels over that of black pepper.

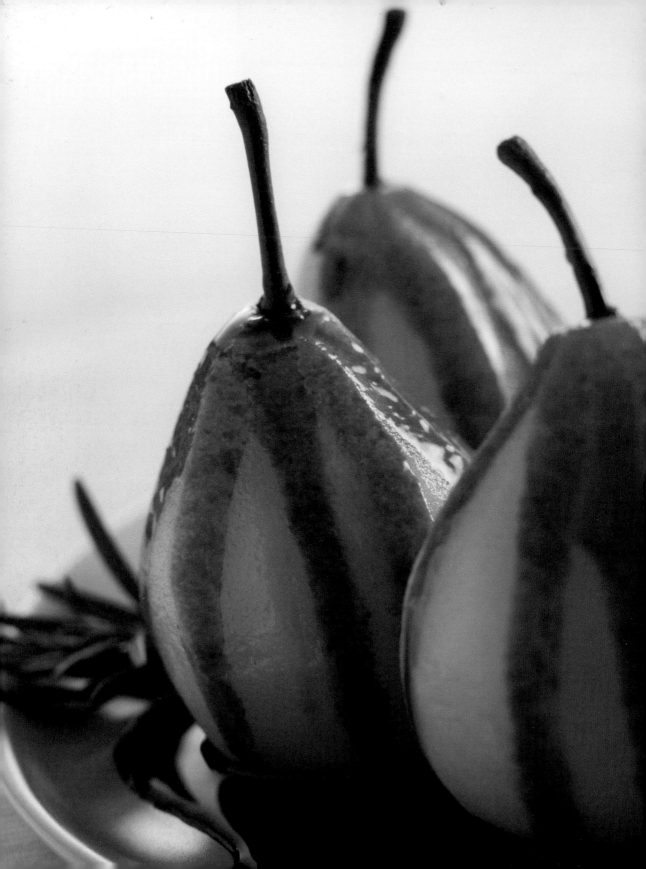

CHAPTER 17

DESSERTS & SNACKS

"The human body is its own best apothecary. The most successful prescriptions are those filled by the body itself."

— NORMAN COUSINS

A s you begin to eat a more healthful diet and cleanse and detoxify your body, you'll discover that you'll lose the desire to end your meal with a heavy dessert, especially one that's laden with fat and calories. ("Stressed" is "desserts" spelled backward.) Of course, every so often, everyone craves a luscious treat, and there are even those times when you want to eat something sweet instead of a meal. Well, you're in luck!

I've included a variety of desserts that you can enjoy sharing with your family and friends. Remember, keep your ingredients as pure as possible so that you obtain the maximum health benefits from every meal—even during dessert. In fact, these recipes can double as meals in themselves. (Well, maybe not the Premium Moist & Chewy Brownies, but most of them.) The first recipe in this chapter makes a great lunch. It's so good that it's hard to believe that it's low in fat and chock-full of isoflavones (from the soy), the phytonutrients that may help prevent cancer.

Even if these desserts weren't so healthful, I'd still like them. They're that delicious. And you can enjoy them without guilt, because they're so nutritious.

À vôtre santé (to your health)!

CHOCOLATE-DATE-PEPPERMINT SHAKE & ICE CREAM

I sometimes have this positively heavenly healthful shake for a meal or afternoon snack.

Serves 2–3.

2 cups nonfat vanilla-soy beverage, almond milk, or vanilla hemp milk
   (see Chapter 2)
1 large or 2 small ripe frozen bananas
5–6 medjool dates, pitted and chopped
4–5 ice cubes
2 Tbsp. cocoa powder
⅛ tsp. peppermint extract

The Shake: Place all ingredients in a blender and blend until creamy smooth, about 60–90 seconds.

The Ice Cream: Follow the steps for the shake, then pour the shake into ice-cube trays. After the cubes are frozen, press them through a Champion Juicer to create a delicious ice cream, although the ice actually makes it more like a sorbet. For a creamier texture, omit the ice cubes and add one more frozen banana and one more date, or use a regular vanilla beverage instead of nonfat. After pressing the frozen cubes through your juicer, you'll have a delicious chocolate-date-peppermint ice cream. Try enjoying it with a pressed frozen banana. Serve in chilled bowls.

Variations: Instead of peppermint extract, substitute orange. Or try it without any extract. You even can include some fresh peppermint or spearmint. To add more nutrients (and protein) to the shake or ice cream, add 1 heaping Tbsp. protein powder. You can also pour coconut milk into ice-cube trays and freeze. Press them through a Champion Juicer together with the ice-cream cubes for a delicious combination.

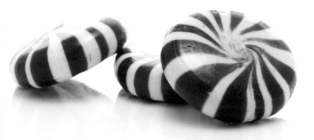

FROZEN-FRUIT TREATS

Here's another simple way to get more fresh fruit into your diet. It's hard to believe that these delicious desserts are actually very good for you.
Serves 2.

2 cups of your favorite fruit, frozen (blueberries, strawberries, pitted black
    cherries, mangos, papayas, raspberries, apricots, or bananas)
Fresh fruit juices such as apple, orange, or pineapple
Fresh mint sprigs

In a blender or food processor, blend your favorite frozen fruit until smooth, adding just enough freshly squeezed juice so that it blends well. Serve immediately in chilled bowls, or freeze for one hour to increase firmness before serving. Garnish with mint sprigs.
Variations: When you're blending any of these fruit ices, try adding a couple drops of pure organic extracts: peppermint, orange, almond, vanilla, or lemon to vary the flavors.

APPLE-WALNUT PUDDING

The combination of apple and walnut always evokes happy feelings for me.
Serves 3–6.

2 cups dried apples, soaked for 8 hours in 4 cups of purified water
    (save the water)
1 apple, peeled, cored, and finely chopped
1 cup raw walnuts, soaked for 8 hours in 2 cups of purified water
4 drops liquid Stevia (a natural sweetener that you can find at your
    natural-food store)
1 ripe banana
Cinnamon to taste

In a food processor or blender, purée all ingredients along with the water from soaking the apples. Chill in the refrigerator. Serve cold.

RAW SUNFLOWER-APRICOT COOKIES

Simply delicious, and so very good for you, too.
Serves 6–8.

3 cups raw sunflower seeds, soaked in purified water overnight or for 8 hours
1 cup raisins, soaked overnight or for 8 hours
1 cup unsulfured dried apricots, chopped and soaked overnight
½ cup raw cashew butter
½ cup raw almond butter
1 Tbsp. pure vanilla extract
1 tsp. almond extract
½ tsp. cinnamon
⅛ tsp. pure organic orange extract

After soaking the apricots, sunflower seeds, and raisins, drain and spread them out on two clean, dry dish towels to remove any extra moisture. In a food processor, blend all ingredients into a nutty consistency. Transfer to a large bowl. Make equal-size small balls, 1" to 1½" in diameter. Press out to ¼-inch thickness. Cover and refrigerate for 1–2 hours before serving. If you can, try making them in a low-temperature dehydrator. (See the Resources section for ordering information.) The cookies come out a little crispy, but they still retain all of the live enzymes and vital nutrients.

DRIED-PLUM & CHOCOLATE WHIP

"Dried plum" is a fancy way of saying *prune,* but don't let that word cause you to turn the page too quickly. You'll love this light, melt-in-your-mouth dessert.
Serves 2–3.

1⅔ cups pitted stewed prunes
2 oz. organic silken tofu
2 Tbsp. cocoa powder
2 Tbsp. pure maple syrup

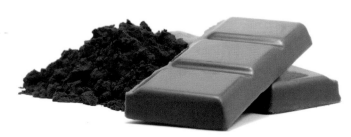

Pour boiling water over prunes, cover, and let stand for 2 hours. Save the stewing liquid to use when blending. Or you can buy stewed prunes, without preservatives, in a can. In a blender or food processor, purée all ingredients together using just enough of the saved cooking liquid to create a creamy, smooth consistency. Chill and serve.

Variations: Instead of the cocoa powder, substitute carob powder and try adding ⅛ tsp. peppermint or orange extract.

FYI: Prunes (Dried Plums)

Prunes, which are really dried plums, are a powerhouse of both insoluble and soluble fiber. In addition, they're an excellent laxative and help lower cholesterol. They provide a healthful dose of magnesium, calcium, potassium, beta-carotene, and iron, too. Studies reveal that ½ cup of prune juice or 3 prunes a day is all it takes to establish regularity. Make sure the fruit is free of preservatives.

Besides being stewed, prunes can be chopped and added to cereal or salads as well as to grain dishes. In fact, chopped prunes can be substituted for raisins in almost any recipe. Finally, if you purée the stewed prunes in their stewing liquid, you can use this purée in recipes for baked goods in place of eggs or most of the oil. It helps bind the ingredients together and keeps them moist.

CINNAMON-VANILLA POACHED PEARS

This elegant dessert wins rave reviews at dinner parties or family gatherings. It's so easy and healthfully delicious—a winning combination.

Serves 4–8.

4 Anjou or Bosc pears, peeled, cored, and cut in half (I prefer them unpeeled)
1 cup apple juice
½ cup purified water
1 (3-inch) piece vanilla bean, cut in half lengthwise
1 (1- to 2-inch) piece cinnamon stick
1 Tbsp. pure maple syrup
Mint sprig

In a large skillet, combine the water and apple juice, maple syrup, and cinnamon stick. With a knife, scrape the seeds from the vanilla bean into the water, then add the bean pods, too. (Save the rest of the bean.) Over medium heat, bring the liquid to a simmer for about 3 minutes so that the vanilla flavor permeates the liquid. Add the pear halves to the liquid, core side up. Spoon some of the poaching liquid into the core cavity. Cover and continue to simmer gently until the pears are tender, about 8–10 minutes. Cool in the liquid, then chill the pears in the refrigerator. To serve, place 1 or 2 pear halves in a bowl and top with some poaching liquid and a sprig of fresh mint.

FYI: Pears

There are more than 3,000 varieties of pears, but only a handful are commercially popular. Perhaps the oldest cultivated fruit in the world, pears aid digestion, are an excellent source of fiber, and provide vitamin C and iron. Bartletts are juicy, tasty, and yellow in color; Comice are red-blushed yellow and not quite as juicy; Bosc are less juicy and more chewy with a russet skin; and Anjou are yellow-green and the only variety that will ripen in the refrigerator. Always choose firm, well-shaped pears that are free of bruises and soft spots.

STRAWBERRY-MANGO-BANANA ICE CREAM

Everyone loves this dessert, and you can make it in seconds.
Serves 2–3.

1 very ripe mango, diced
8 large frozen strawberries
2 large frozen bananas, cut into chunks

In a blender or food processor, blend the mango. Add the strawberries and bananas until the consistency becomes just like ice cream. Serve in chilled bowls.

Tip: Frozen Bananas

Use ripe (spotted) bananas. They're sweeter, easier to digest, and more flavorful. Peel and freeze whole in a zip-top freezer bag. Press out extra air before locking shut to prevent browning. I keep a dozen or two on hand so that they're readily available for fruit ice cream and smoothies.

SESAME-BANANA-ORANGE PUDDING

If you thought pudding wasn't good for you, here's an easy 2-minute recipe that will change your mind.

Serves 1.

1 ripe banana
1 large medjool date, chopped
2 Tbsp. raw sesame seeds
2 drops pure organic orange extract
Dash cinnamon

In a blender or food processor, blend the banana and date together. In a nut grinder, grind the sesame seeds to create a meal. Add the sesame-seed meal and the orange extract to the banana-and-date mixture and blend. Serve in a small chilled bowl. Garnish with a dash of cinnamon.

Variations: You can blend a few seconds longer and add a teaspoon of pure maple syrup, if you like it sweeter. Instead of sesame seeds, try 1½ Tbsp. raw tahini.

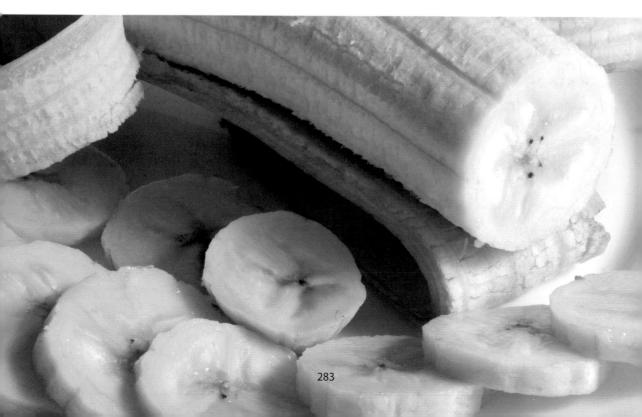

OUTRAGEOUS OATMEAL COOKIES

Since these scrumptious cookies freeze well, you might want to make extra so that you have them on hand for unexpected guests or for special treats.
Makes 20–24 cookies.

2 cups oat flour (I make it fresh in my kitchen mill; see the Resources section
    for ordering information)
2 cups rolled oats
1 cup apple juice
½ cup raisins
⅓ cup flaxseed meal
2 ripe bananas
⅓ cup applesauce
1 Tbsp. frozen apple-juice concentrate
½ tsp. baking soda
1 tsp. baking powder
1 tsp. cinnamon
¼ tsp. nutmeg

Preheat oven to 375° F. In a large bowl, combine the oat flour, rolled oats, flaxseed meal, baking soda, baking powder, and spices. In a blender or food processor, purée the bananas, juice, concentrate, and applesauce. Add the dry mixture to the apple mixture a little at a time, while mixing. Stir in the raisins. Drop by spoonfuls on a nonstick baking sheet. Bake in the center of the oven for about 10–12 minutes. (Make sure not to overbake!)

Variations: Add unsweetened dried cherries and/or shredded coconut instead of the raisins. You can also use unfrozen apple-juice concentrate, which you can find in a glass jar in most natural-food stores and many regular supermarkets.

Tip: Excalibur Food Dehydrator

Whether making dried fruit, veggie chips, cookies, granola, crackers, burgers, fruit leathers, etc., I use and recommend the Excalibur Food Dehydrator. To order, see page 327. Visit: **www.dry123.com.**

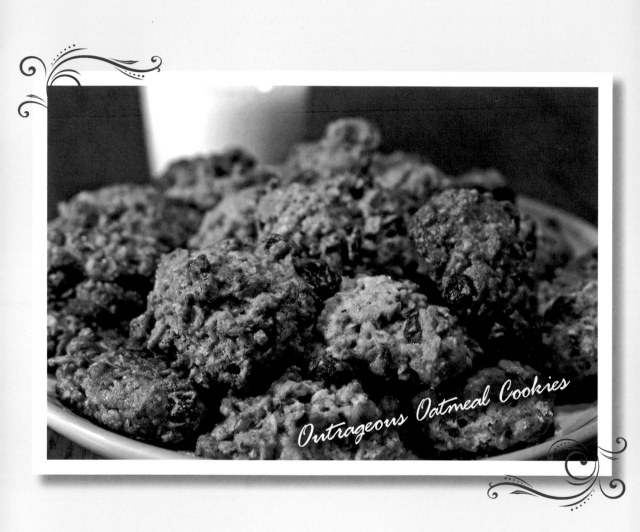

Outrageous Oatmeal Cookies

FYI: Oats & Oat Bran

Oats and oat bran are excellent sources of soluble fiber, which is the kind that helps lower cholesterol. Oatmeal, also called rolled oats, is available as regular (or old fashioned), which cooks in about 15 minutes, and quick cooking, which takes about 5 minutes. Instant oatmeal requires almost no cooking, but it's hard to find it without added sugar or salt. Steel-cut, or Scotch, oats (my favorite) can take 45 minutes to an hour to cook. They have a nuttier flavor and consistency. If you've never tried them, get some soon and try my Oatmeal Deluxe recipe in Chapter 3.

THE BEST APPLE-BERRY SAUCE

I keep lots of this yummy sauce on hand to eat as a snack between meals. You also can use it in baked goods. It reduces the need for oil and other fats and keeps cakes and breads nice and moist.

Serves 6–8.

6–8 apples, your favorite variety (mine is Fuji)
1½ cups freshly squeezed apple juice (or water or both)
1 cup blueberries, strawberries, or raspberries (or combination)
4 tsp. concentrated fruit sweetener, such as apple, berry, or black cherry
1 tsp. cinnamon
¼ tsp. lemon zest (from an organic lemon only)
¼ tsp. orange zest (from an organic orange only)
2 dates, pitted and chopped

Core and chop the apples (if they're not organic, peel them first). In a large saucepan, bring the juice (or water) to a boil and add the apples. Cover and return to a boil, then lower the heat and simmer for about 10 minutes. Drain. Set aside to cool. Place cooked apples in a food processor along with the berries and purée. Add concentrated fruit sweetener, dates, and spices and pulse until you get the consistency you like best. Keep refrigerated in an airtight container. Try this applesauce over fresh fruit, whole-grain pancakes, or oatmeal, or spread on whole-grain toast.

FYI: Apples

Apples are the perfect health and diet food. They elevate your blood-glucose level safely and gently, and then keep it up for a longer period of time than apple juice or sweeter fruits, such as bananas or grapes, so you feel fuller longer. Apples have abundant soluble fiber, which helps stabilize blood-sugar levels and guards against sudden drops in energy or mood swings. They have virtually no sodium, saturated fat, or cholesterol. In fact, according to studies at Yale University, apples help reduce the level of cholesterol in your blood and also lower blood pressure. I guess the old 19th-century apple advertisement is true: "An apple a day keeps the doctor away."

CASHEW-RAISIN BALLS

These freeze beautifully, so double or triple the batch to keep on hand as the perfect treat or snack to satisfy a sweet tooth. They're much better for you than M&M's!

Makes about 3½ cups.

1 cup raisins, soaked overnight in purified water, drained, and dried
1 lb. whole raw cashews (or almonds or walnuts)
¼ cup rolled oats
12 dates, pitted
3 Tbsp. raw tahini
2 Tbsp. shredded coconut
1 tsp. cinnamon
1 tsp. pure vanilla extract

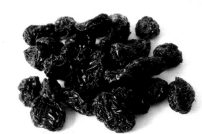

In a blender or food processor, finely grind cashews and oats together. Transfer to a bowl. In a blender, combine the dates, tahini, coconut, cinnamon, and vanilla. Add the raisins and pulse until all is mixed. Combine mixture with oats, then roll into balls. They can be as small as 1 inch or as large as 2 inches in diameter. Store in the refrigerator, or freeze for later use.

FYI: Cashews

Cashews are higher in calories than many other plant foods, but they're lower in fat than most other nuts. They're also rich in calcium, magnesium, iron, zinc, and folic acid.

NUT-DATE BALLS

Ask your children to help you make these delicious treats. They make terrific gifts (if you can keep from eating all of them yourself).

Serves 6–8.

½ cup raw cashews
½ cup raw almonds
¼ cup raw walnuts
¼ cup flaxseed meal
½ cup chopped dried, unsulfured black figs
1 cup chopped dates, preferably medjool
Unsweetened shredded coconut
Raw sesame seeds
Raw hemp nuts

In a food processor, blender, or nut grinder, grind the nuts (except the hemp nuts, which are already small) into a meal. Add flaxseed meal. Add the chopped fruit and blend until well mixed. Roll into balls about the diameter of a quarter, then roll the balls in the coconut, sesame seeds, or hemp nuts. These freeze well, so consider making extra so you have them on hand. These also make great snacks.

Variations: You also can add a little raw nut or seed butter (such as almond, sunflower, pumpkin, hemp, tahini, or cashew) to the mixture. For a real treat, incorporate some raw chocolate nibs or raw cocoa powder with some agave nectar to sweeten them a tad more.

PREMIUM MOIST & CHEWY CHOCOLATE BROWNIES

You won't miss the butter, sugar, eggs, or other animal fat in these moist and luscious brownies. This recipe and the one that follows are equally delicious and will garner rave reviews. You can make them in a glass or metal pan or in a muffin tin. I like using a mini-muffin tin for smaller treats, as well as a heart-shaped muffin tin.

Serves 12.

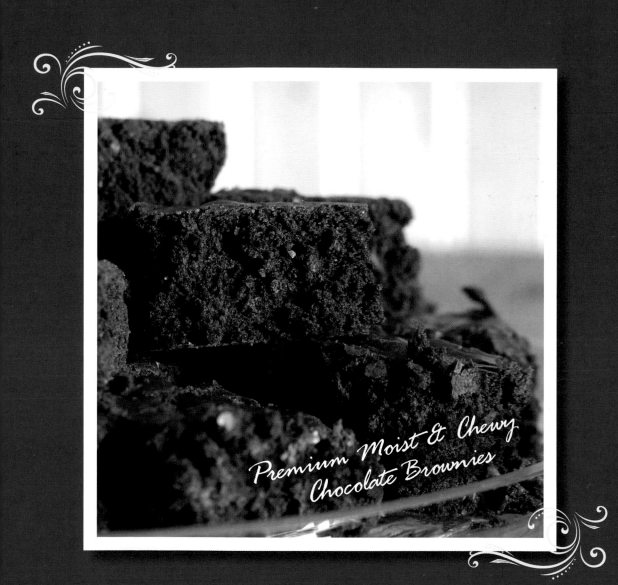

Premium Moist & Chewy
Chocolate Brownies

1 cup oat flour (I make this fresh with my kitchen mill; see the
     Resources section for ordering information)
⅔ cup cocoa powder
2 Tbsp. arrowroot
½ tsp. baking soda
2 tsp. baking powder
⅛ tsp. sea salt
¾ cup unsweetened applesauce
⅓ cup chopped walnuts
⅓ cup plus 2 Tbsp. agave nectar
⅓ cup pitted, chopped dates
¼ cup raisins
1 tsp. vanilla extract
Nonstick cooking spray

Preheat oven to 350° F. Mix together the dry ingredients in a medium bowl. Combine wet ingredients and add to the dry mixture, stirring thoroughly. Spoon batter into an 8" x 8" glass or metal baking pan coated with nonstick cooking spray. Bake in preheated oven 25 to 30 minutes. For mini muffins: bake 10 to 12 minutes. For regular-size muffins: bake 12 to15 minutes. Test with a toothpick for doneness.

Each brownie square or muffin has 90 calories, 15 grams of carbohydrate, and 5 grams of fiber.

DOUBLE CHOCOLATE OMEGA BROWNIES

With this recipe and the preceding one, I usually quadruple the ingredients and make lots of extra mini-muffin brownies because they freeze so well. And when you have the desire for just a touch of delicious chocolate that's good for you to boot, these mini muffins hit the spot. In fact, they're delicious popped into your mouth right out of the freezer!

Serves 12.

1 cup oat flour (I make this fresh with my kitchen mill; see the
     Resources section for ordering information)
½ cup cocoa powder
2 Tbsp. arrowroot

½ tsp. baking soda
2 tsp. baking powder
⅛ tsp. sea salt
⅓ cup chopped walnuts
⅓ cup pitted, chopped dates
½ cup unsweetened applesauce
¼ cup raisins
⅓ cup agave nectar
¼ cup chocolate hemp milk (I recommend
    Living Harvest Hemp Milk, rich in omega-3s)
1 tsp. vanilla extract
Nonstick cooking spray

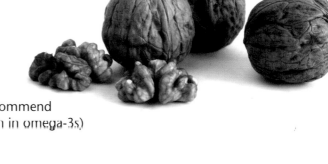

Preheat oven to 350° F. Mix together the dry ingredients in a medium bowl. Combine wet ingredients and add to the dry mixture, stirring thoroughly. Pour into an 8" x 8" glass or metal baking pan, or a muffin tin coated with a nonstick cooking spray. Bake in a preheated oven for 25 to 30 minutes for the 8" x 8" pan, 10 to 12 minutes if using a mini-muffin pan, and 12 to 15 minutes if using a regular-size muffin pan. Test for doneness with a toothpick.

Each brownie square or muffin has 90 calories, 13 grams of carbohydrate, and 5 grams of fiber.

FYI: Chocolate

Chocolate, which is native to tropical Central America, was believed to be a food of the gods, and I can see why! In Mexico as late as 1885, cocoa beans were used as standard currency. Once the beans are removed from the pods of the cacao tree, they're roasted, chopped up, and ground into an oily paste called "chocolate mass" or "liquor." The liquor is suspended in the cocoa butter, which is more than 50 percent fatty acids. To make powder, most of the cocoa butter is pressed out of the liquor.

The taste of chocolate depends upon the variety of the cacao tree, the soil it was grown in, and what it's blended with, as well as the processing. Bitter chocolate is a diuretic and an antioxidant. The darker chocolate has more antioxidants, and white has none. Chocolate may help lower blood pressure and is even considered to be an aphrodisiac. It's said to release the brain chemicals responsible for the feeling of being in love. While it may have some benefits, keep in mind that it also contains theobromine, which, like caffeine, can trigger various nervous symptoms, including insomnia, hyperactivity in children, anxiety, and mood swings. When I eat chocolate, I try to choose organically grown cocoa beans and dark chocolate, which has no dairy added. I also use raw chocolate powder, nibs, and other raw sources more than heated varieties.

CRACKER-JACK POPCORN

A healthful variation on an old snack favorite.
Makes about 5 cups.

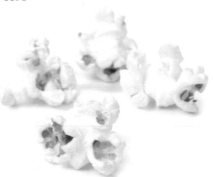

3½ cups air-popped popcorn
⅔ cup raw cashew pieces or hemp nuts (optional)
⅓ cup barley-malt syrup
⅓ cup rice syrup
½ tsp. sea salt
Nonstick cooking spray

Preheat oven to 300° F. In a saucepan, heat the barley-malt and rice syrups and sea salt together until they're hot, but not boiling. In a large bowl, mix the popcorn and nuts, then pour the syrup mixture over them. Mix by hand, being sure to lightly oil your hands first (this is sticky stuff). On a large nonstick baking sheet that's been sprayed with nonstick cooking spray, spread out the corn mixture and bake until lightly crisp, about 5 minutes. Watch it carefully to be sure it doesn't burn.

TAPIOCA PUDDING WITH TOASTED ALMONDS

Here's a healthful alternative to store-bought tapioca.
Serves 3–4.

2 cups vanilla rice milk
½ cup tapioca
⅓ cup chopped almonds, toasted in a dry skillet
¼ cup maple syrup
½ tsp. pure almond extract
⅛ tsp. sea salt

In a medium saucepan without heat, combine the rice milk, tapioca, syrup, and salt. Stir the mixture and let it stand for 5 minutes. Then bring it to a full boil over medium heat, stirring constantly. Remove from the heat and stir in almond extract. Pour into 3–4 dessert cups. Sprinkle toasted nuts over pudding mixture. Serve warm or cold.

FROZEN COCONUT-BERRY-MINT PIE

This mouthwatering pie is the very best way to introduce raw food to family and friends.

Serves 6–8.

The Crust:
1 Tbsp. carob or cocoa powder (I use raw cocoa powder)
1 cup walnuts
1 cup almonds
1 cup unsweetened shredded coconut
¾ cup apple juice
⅓ cup fresh flaxseed meal
¼ tsp. pure organic peppermint extract
2 Tbsp. apple-juice concentrate

The Filling:
4 cups fresh or frozen berries (blueberries, strawberries, blackberries, or raspberries)
3 oz. soft lite organic silken tofu (not a raw food)
6 medjool dates, pitted and sliced
½ cup lite coconut milk
1 Tbsp. apple-juice concentrate
¼ tsp. pure organic peppermint extract

To make the crust: Place all of the ingredients in a blender or food processor and blend to combine. Transfer to a glass pie dish and use your hands to spread the mixture evenly across the bottom and sides. Refrigerate.

To make the filling: Place all of the ingredients in a blender or food processor and purée until creamy smooth. Pour into the chilled crust and smooth it with a spatula or knife. Cover and freeze until firm, at least 2 hours.

Variation: To create a tropical pie, use a combination of fresh or frozen pineapple, mango, and papaya.

FYI: Berries

With an average of 50 calories per ½ cup, berries are a perfect weight-loss food. Whether served fresh in a bowl; added to smoothies; or made into fruit ices, sorbets, ice cream, or pies, it's hard to resist these colorful, delectable fruits. They're full of fiber and potassium and enough natural fructose to satisfy any craving for sweets.

GINGER-FRUIT SALAD

Fresh ginger juice and lemon zest give this fruit salad a wonderful zip. Serves 3–4.

2 apples, peeled, cored, and chopped
1 orange, peeled and seeded
1 ripe banana, sliced
1 ripe pear, peeled, cored, and chopped
1 cup strawberries or other berry in season, stemmed and chopped
1 Tbsp. maple syrup
½ tsp. fresh lemon zest (from an organic lemon only)
1½ tsp. fresh ginger juice
Fresh mint sprigs

In a blender or food processor, purée the orange, maple syrup, lemon zest, and ginger juice. In a bowl, combine the rest of the fruit, toss with the purée, and chill before serving. Garnish with fresh mint sprigs.

FYI: Ginger

Rich in calcium, magnesium, phosphorus, and potassium, ginger helps prevent nausea, is good for menstrual cramps, and helps improve circulation. A favorite of gourmet chefs, this root is such a versatile food that it can be juiced, sautéed, puréed, stir-fried, and simply made into a soothing tea when a sliver is mixed with some hot water and fresh lemon. That's what I start each day with—lemon-ginger water. I also like to add a thin sliver of fresh ginger root to other organic teas such as peppermint, chamomile, rose-hip, or green tea.

APPLE-LEMON CRISP

It's hard to believe that something this sweet and tasty is good for you.
Serves 5–6.

Filling:
2½ pounds Granny Smith apples (about 5–6), peeled or unpeeled
    (which I prefer), cored, and cut into ½-inch-thick slices
¾ cup golden raisins
⅓ cup sugar-free orange marmalade
1 small organic lemon

Topping:
1 cup rolled oats
⅓ cup maple-syrup granules
⅓ cup chopped almonds
¼ cup unbleached all-purpose flour
¼ cup Smart Balance (an alternative to butter or margarine), chilled
1 Tbsp. fresh flaxseed meal
1 tsp. sesame seeds
⅛ tsp. sea salt
⅛ tsp. cinnamon
Nonstick cooking spray

Preheat oven to 375° F. Use an 8" square baking dish and spray with nonstick cooking spray. In a bowl, combine apple slices, raisins, and marmalade so that the apples are completely coated. Take half the filling and arrange in the baking dish. Cut the lemon into thin slices, discarding the ends and seeds. Cut slices in half and arrange over the apple filling to cover most of the apples. Top with the rest of the apple mixture.

In a nut grinder, grind the sesame seeds and flaxseed for 10 seconds to create meal. In a bowl, combine the oats, flour, maple granules, cinnamon, nuts, sesame seed, flaxseed meal, and salt. Mix in the Smart Balance spread, trying to moisten all of the flour and oats. Spread this mixture evenly over the apple filling. Bake about 50 minutes, or until the topping is lightly browned and firm. Let stand for 30 minutes, and serve it warm.

Variations: Substitute regular raisins or dried cherries for the golden raisins; use chopped walnuts, cashews, or hazelnuts for the almonds, and peaches, nectarines, mangos, papayas, or blueberries in place of the apples. Substitute apricot, blueberry, raspberry, peach, or strawberry sugar-free jams for the marmalade, and top with fruit ice cream. You can also use your own granola in place of the oats.

TROPICAL SORBET

On a hot summer day, this sorbet will have you jumping for joy.

Serves 3–4.

2 cups pineapple chunks, frozen
3 frozen strawberries
1 ripe banana
¼ cup lite coconut milk
2 Tbsp. orange juice

In a food processor or blender, purée the pineapple, banana, and strawberries while slowly adding the juice and coconut milk. Stop occasionally and scrape down the sides. Blend until smooth. Spoon into dessert cups and freeze for 1 hour before serving.

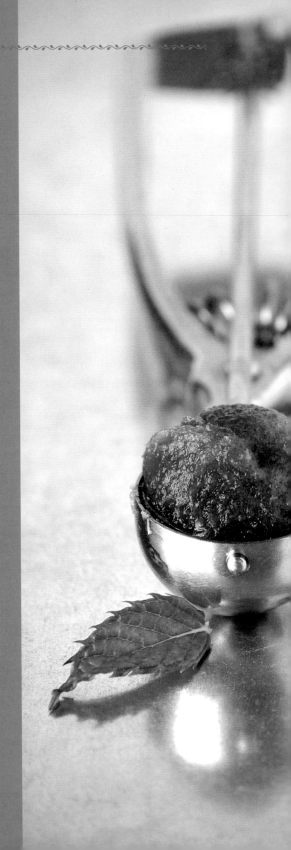

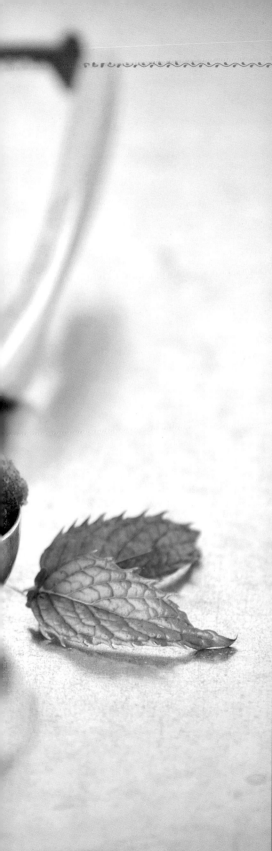

CAROB FROZEN-BANANA STICKS

This is one of those recipes you'll want to double or triple so that the sticks are always available for a healthful dessert or snack.
Serves 4.

4 firm small bananas
⅔ cup raw carob powder
½–⅔ cup purified water
⅛ tsp. pure organic peppermint extract
4 Popsicle sticks

Place a stick in each peeled banana. Warm the water to 107–108° F, but no hotter, so that you can keep this treat vitally alive. Add the peppermint oil and stir. Add the carob powder and mix until dissolved. Dip each banana in the carob mixture. Use a deep enough container to cover the banana—you can spoon or brush it on the areas needing extra. Wrap each coated banana in a piece of waxed paper and freeze overnight. They'll keep for 1–2 months in your freezer.

FYI: Carob

Carob, also referred to as Saint John's bread, is the leguminous pod of the locust tree and approximates the taste of chocolate. Roasted and ground pods yield carob powder. Sweet, light, and dry, carob is alkaline in nature. It does contain tannin (as does cocoa), which reduces the absorption of protein through the intestinal wall, so use it as a special treat rather than daily fare. Carob is an excellent source of calcium, containing more than 3 times as much as milk. It's also rich in potassium and other nutrients. It has less fat and fewer calories than chocolate; and unlike chocolate, it's naturally sweet, with almost 50 percent sugar, and is free of caffeine and oxalic acids.

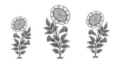

CHAPTER 18

MEALS KIDS LOVE

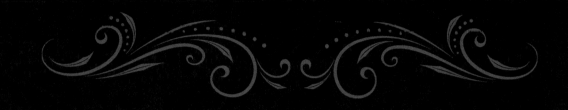

"Your imagination is your preview of life's coming attractions."

— ALBERT EINSTEIN

Although this chapter is geared toward great foods to serve kids, you don't have to be a little one to enjoy them. Experiment and add your own special touches to make them work even better for your entire family.

As I discussed earlier, healthful eating and exercise are fundamental ingredients for a healthy childhood. Every parent faces a bewildering array of choices, each championed by an avalanche of misinformation from the food industry. How can you ensure that your children eat right?

Fortunately, the dietary principles you need to understand are relatively simple (and they're the same ones that should guide *your* choices, too). Make sure your children eat as many leafy-green and other vegetables as possible and that they consume enough extra calories from fruits, beans, grains, nuts, seeds, and avocados so that they don't get too skinny. Encourage them to avoid the typical high-sugar, high-fat, low-nutrient diet that's leading to the epidemic of childhood obesity.

All of the recipes that follow are healthful and delicious, and your children will enjoy them!

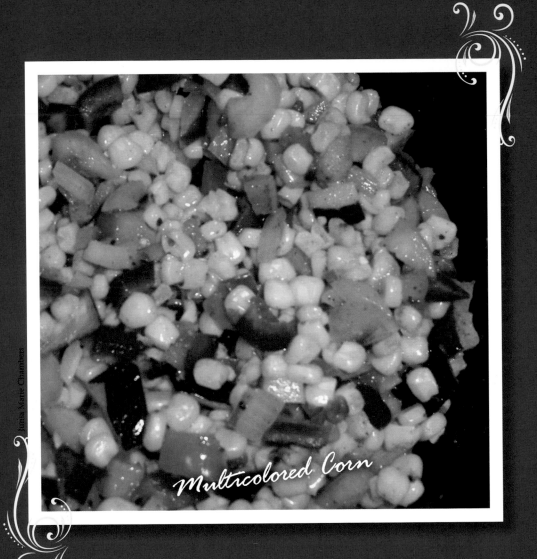

Multicolored Corn

Junita Marie Chambers

SWEET-POTATO HOME FRIES

Here's a sweet, healthful, baked treat kids love. But let me warn you: You'll run out of these fast, so you might consider quadrupling the recipe.
Serves 2–4.

2 large sweet potatoes/yams, scrubbed and cut into 1" x 3" "fries"
2 Tbsp. cold-pressed, extra-virgin olive oil
Sea salt to taste

Preheat oven to 450° F. Arrange sweet potatoes on a baking sheet and drizzle oil all over them to coat. Sprinkle with salt. Bake for 15 minutes, then broil for about 10 minutes, gently turning over after 5 minutes. (My local market sells precut sweet potatoes to make into fries. Maybe yours does, too.)

Variation 1: If you have a spray-pump bottle, try spritzing the fries with olive oil mixed with low-sodium tamari instead of using the salt. The light mist gives a more evenly applied coating with less fat. Use cinnamon and maple syrup instead of oil for sweeter fries. Try sprinkling on your favorite herbs such as rosemary or chives, or use garlic or onion powder. For an earthier treat, try cinnamon, nutmeg, and allspice.

Variation 2: Dip each sliced potato into a bowl of broth and bake, or use ⅔ cup coconut water from young coconuts. You can purchase the young coconuts in the natural-food store and cut the tops off yourself (although this is difficult without the best knife). You also can find the water already removed from the coconut in the refrigerator section, or even in unrefrigerated cartons.

MULTICOLORED CORN

Kids love corn! For this festive and colorful vegetable dish, all you need to do is some chopping; the rest comes together in minutes.
Serves 4–6.

2½ cups fresh whole corn kernels
⅓ cup finely chopped red bell pepper
⅓ cup finely chopped orange bell pepper
⅓ cup finely chopped yellow bell pepper

⅓ cup finely chopped purple bell pepper
½ cup minced sweet onion (such as Vidalia or Maui)
⅓ cup finely chopped green onion
1 clove garlic, minced
1 tsp. cold-pressed, extra-virgin olive oil
½ tsp. ground cinnamon
Sea salt to taste

In a nonstick skillet, heat the oil, then add sweet and green onions and garlic. Sauté for 2 minutes. Add all remaining ingredients and stir briefly. Add salt to taste if desired, then cover and cook over low heat about 3–4 minutes, stirring often.

FLAVORFUL RICE PILAF

Don't let the long list of ingredients daunt you. If you have everything on hand, this can be prepared with little effort.
Serves 4–6.

1½ cups purified water
½ cup coconut water or lite coconut milk
1 cup uncooked basmati rice
1 cup grated carrots
½ cup unsweetened shredded coconut
½ cup frozen green peas, thawed
⅓ cup frozen sweet corn, thawed
2 Tbsp. sesame seeds
4 Tbsp. slivered almonds
2 Tbsp. raisin or currants
2 Tbsp. pitted dates, chopped
1 Tbsp. cold-pressed sesame oil
5 whole cloves
4 cardamom pods
1 tsp. sea salt
¼ tsp. ground cinnamon
Unsalted roasted pistachio nuts

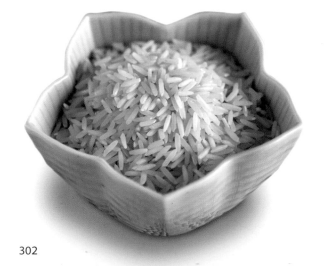

In a large saucepan, heat the water and coconut water or milk. In a skillet over medium heat, heat the oil and sauté the shredded coconut, sesame seeds, almonds, cardamom pods, cloves, and cinnamon just until the coconut begins to turn light brown. Rinse the rice and drain. Add rice to the skillet mixture and cook, stirring constantly, for 3–5 minutes.

Bring the water and coconut milk to a boil and add the rice mixture, carrots, raisins, dates, and salt. Stir and return to a boil. Cover, lower the heat, and simmer for 25 minutes or until all of the liquid is absorbed. Turn off the heat and let the rice sit for 10 minutes. Remove the cloves. Add the corn and peas just before serving. Coarsely chop the pistachio nuts and sprinkle on top as a garnish.

Tip: Basmati Rice

Basmati is a delicious, long-grain rice that has a buttery aroma, nutty flavor, and fluffy texture. Available in both whole-grain (brown) and refined-white varieties, each grain almost doubles in length when cooked with little change in thickness. As with all rice, the whole grain is far superior in nutritional value to the refined-white version.

PIZZA PIZZAZZ

This is a great way to get the whole family involved in making the meal. You won't miss the dairy or meat toppings on this sensational pizza.

1–2 per person whole-wheat, fat-free chapatis, tortillas, or
   split whole-grain pita

2 Tbsp. grated jalapeno soy cheese (soy mozzarella or
   any other nondairy cheese)

2 zucchini, cut in half and sliced lengthwise into ¼-inch-thick strips

½ Tbsp. per person chopped green onions

2–3 strips per person roasted red bell peppers
   (see Chapter 16)

½ Tbsp. per person sliced olives

2 Tbsp. per person salsa (see Chapter 4)

2–4 slices per person slices of avocado or Tbsp. of guacamole (see Chapter 4)

Steam zucchini until slightly tender, about 2 minutes. On a baking sheet, toast the flatbread in the oven until crisp but not brown. You can mist it with a dash of olive oil and tamari if you like. Remove from the oven, then preheat the broiler. Cover crusts with a thin layer of salsa followed by the cheese. Then arrange the roasted bell peppers, zucchini, olives, and green onions on the top. Top with more cheese.

Broil for 3–5 minutes away from the heat, or until the cheese melts. Keep an eye on them so that they don't overcook or burn. Remove from the broiler and immediately add a few avocado slices or guacamole. Serve with extra salsa on top.

Variations: In my book *Be Healthy~Stay Balanced,* I offer some recipes for delicious nondairy cheeses, a goat-like cheese, sour cream, and yogurt. These make great toppings, too.

POTATOES ROSÉ WITH EMERALD GREEN GRAVY

The beets turn this potato dish a delightful shade of pink. The green sauce spooned on top is a hit with the kids.
Serves 4–6.

2 lbs. Yukon Gold potatoes, peeled and cut into chunks
¼ cup plain soy, hemp, almond, or cashew milk (see Chapter 2)
1 small beet
2 tsp. minced fresh chives or parsley
1 tsp. sea salt
Emerald Green Sauce (see Chapter 4)

Juice the beet and reserve 3 Tbsp. juice. In a medium saucepan, cover potatoes with water. Bring to a boil, cover, lower heat, and simmer for about 15–20 minutes or until the potatoes are tender, but not mushy. Drain.

In a small saucepan, warm the milk. Mash the potatoes, add the 3 Tbsp. beet juice, and mash to combine. Then add enough milk to create the desired consistency. Add salt to taste and garnish with chives or parsley. Serve immediately with Emerald Green Sauce.

Variations: Use carrot juice for an orange color or substitute half yams or sweet potatoes for half of the Yukon Golds. If your family loves garlic, add roasted garlic when mashing.

SENSATIONAL SPAGHETTI SQUASH

This squash goes well with a mixture of steamed vegetables and a crisp green salad.
Serves 3–4.

½ spaghetti squash, seeded
½ cup grated soy or other cheese
Dash paprika

Place the squash in a large skillet with just enough water to steam without covering the squash. Steam until tender, about 45 minutes. Scoop out the flesh with a fork, forming spaghetti-like strands, and sprinkle with the cheese. Season with paprika and serve hot.

Variation: Top with marinara or pasta sauce.

GRATED SALAD WITH A TWIST OF LEMON

Combining delicious fruits, vegetables, and nuts, this salad will please even the pickiest eaters.
Serves 4.

1 medium carrot, grated
1 small parsnip, grated
½ small beet, grated
½ cup hearts of palm, sliced into ¼-inch pieces
½ cup raisins or currants, rehydrated in hot water
    for a few minutes and drained
⅓ cup walnuts, chopped and toasted
1 Tbsp. fresh lemon juice
⅓ cup favorite soy or other nondairy yogurt such as vanilla, lemon, or peach
1 tsp. maple syrup
Dash cinnamon

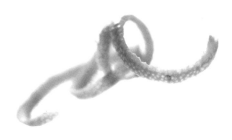

In a large bowl, combine all ingredients. Serve with extra cinnamon lightly sprinkled on top.

FYI: Soy Yogurt

Soy yogurt is a cholesterol- and lactose-free product with a fair approximation of the flavor of dairy yogurt. It's available in all natural-food stores and most supermarkets in a variety of flavors. It has a comparable nutritional profile to soy milk, but has enhanced digestibility because it's fermented.

FAJITAS

You do need to marinate the seitan, so get started on this one early in the day. Once the seitan is marinated, these are quick to prepare and assemble. I usually serve them with guacamole and salsa or a spicy red-chili sauce.

Serves 4–6.

½ lb. seitan (wheat gluten), cut into long strips
1½ cups chopped tomatoes
2 yellow or orange bell peppers, thinly sliced
2 green chilis, chopped (membranes and seeds removed)
1 onion, thinly sliced
1–2 cloves garlic, minced
½ cup mushrooms, sliced
½ tsp. cold-pressed, extra-virgin olive oil
½ cup balsamic vinegar
¼ cup purified water
2 Tbsp. low-sodium tamari
Whole-wheat tortillas

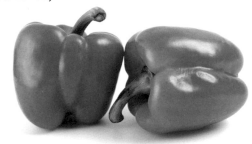

In a large bowl, combine the vinegar, water, tamari, and garlic. Add the seitan and marinate for 3 hours. In a skillet or wok, heat the oil. Add the onions, peppers, and chilis and sauté 7–8 minutes. Add the tomatoes and mushrooms and sauté for 5 minutes. Add the seitan; sauté 7–10 minutes. Warm tortillas in the oven or in a dry skillet, then fill with the seitan mixture and roll them up.

No-Guilt Sweets You Can Feed Your Kids

There's no need to eliminate dessert completely when you have these delicious, healthy recipes. You and your children will love the refreshing, naturally sweet taste of these dishes!

RAW CHERRY-ORANGE APPLESAUCE DELUXE

This fruit sauce can be eaten with a spoon or used over fruit, whole-grain bread or toast, pancakes, waffles, muffins, and crackers. I make double batches weekly, because adults love it as much as kids do.
Serves 2–4.

2 apples, cored and chopped (peeled, if preferred)
1 orange, peeled and sectioned
1–2 dates, pitted
16 Bing cherries, pitted and cut in half
2 Tbsp. fresh apple juice (or water)
½ Tbsp. fresh lemon juice
¼ tsp. cinnamon

In a blender or food processor, combine all ingredients and pulse until a sauce texture is created. Refrigerate before serving.
Variations: When berries are in season (late spring through summer in the U.S.), add your favorites: blueberries, strawberries, raspberries, or blackberries.

MUESLI PARFAIT

Layered into a parfait glass, this crunchy and refreshing treat looks especially appealing to kids.

Serves 3–4.

1 cup muesli or granola (see Chapter 3)
1 cup favorite soy yogurt such as blueberry, strawberry, apple, or kiwi lime
1 cup fresh fruit, sliced
1 cup all-fruit preserves or applesauce
Fresh mint

In a parfait glass, alternately layer yogurt, sliced fruit, preserves, and muesli or granola. Garnish with fresh mint.

STUFFED DATES

I make these monthly and quadruple the recipe. They freeze well, make great gifts, and are convenient to have on hand for unexpected company.

Serves 3–6.

12–14 medjool dates
½ cup almond, sunflower, or cashew butter
Whole raw pecans, cashews, or almonds (one to stuff into each date)
½ cup almonds, pecans, or walnuts (or all of them) to grind into a meal

Split each date with a small, sharp knife, and remove the pit. Press the dates open as you would baked potatoes. Stuff each date with nut butter and a whole almond, pecan, or cashew. You can make each one different, as you'd find in a box of candy. Then close each one up by pinching with your fingers. In a blender, grind almonds, pecans, or walnuts (or a combination) into a meal. Transfer to a shallow bowl. Roll each stuffed date in the nut meal, arrange on a plate or tray, and refrigerate before serving.

Variations: Add some flaxseed meal to the ground nuts to increase the omega-3s. Keep a supply of organic nut and seed butters on hand to add as desired.

FYI: Dates

As the date dries, its fructose changes to sucrose, so the drier the fruit, the sweeter it is. Dates are 60–75 percent sugar, so they're not recommended for people with diabetes, obesity, yeast infections, or respiratory infections. However, they're also rich in fiber and are good sources of iron, niacin, and potassium. Dates can be used to sweeten baked goods, smoothies, granola, puddings, spreads, and sauces. My favorite soft dates, medjools, are allowed to sun dry on the tree and are then hydrated with steam to plump them back up. Try to find organic dates to avoid the pesticide residues found on commercially grown fruits.

Date sugar is made from 100 percent pitted dehydrated dates that are coarsely ground, so it contains all of the nutrients of dried dates. Used in moderation, it's a high-quality sweetener—certainly more natural and unrefined than most. You can sprinkle it on top of cereal or yogurt or add it to baked goods or smoothies. I also rehydrate dates and then purée them with some of the soaking liquid; I use this purée as a sweetener and to enhance moisture in baked goods.

HEALTHFUL CANDY BALLS

For this one, I intentionally omitted any specific measurements so that you could have fun experimenting with the ingredients. Kids love to help make these, so get the whole family involved and make lots of extra. You can freeze them and then pull them out any time for unexpected guests, for a quick snack, or when a sweet craving hits. They're even great frozen!

Raw sunflower seeds
Raw sesame seeds
Raisins
Favorite dried fruit, such as dates or cherries
Apple butter
Pure maple syrup
Pinch of sea salt
Toasted, shredded coconut

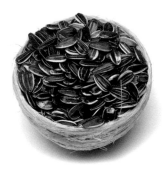

In a food processor, grind together the seeds and dried fruit. Add a little maple syrup, apple butter, and salt. Process until it forms a cohesive ball. (Add more apple butter or syrup if needed.) Section pieces and roll into small balls, about 1½ inch in diameter. Roll these small balls in the shredded coconut.

Variations: Add in some freshly ground flaxseed, cashews, almonds, walnuts, or other favorite nut.

GUILT-FREE BANANA SPLIT

Here's a way to eat a banana split without all of the fat and calories. Makes 1.

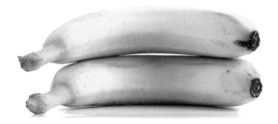

1 banana
½ cup low-fat soy or other nondairy yogurt
3–4 strawberries, sliced
¼ cup diced fresh pineapple
1 Tbsp. chopped pecans and walnuts
1 or 2 fresh pitted cherries

Slice the banana lengthwise and spoon the yogurt between the halves. Top with the strawberries, pineapple, pecans, and walnuts. Top with a fresh cherry or two.

FYI: Bananas

You might not think of bananas as a diet food, but think again. They combat hunger pangs and leave you satisfied and feeling full. It's the combination of fiber and fructose (natural sugar) that gives them their superfood status. The fructose is encased in fiber and carbohydrate so it satisfies a sweet tooth, but releases into your system slowly. In addition to being rich in the mineral potassium, which makes bananas good for hypertension, they're also richer in other minerals than any soft fruit except strawberries. (They have twice as much vitamin C as apples.) Under-ripe or green bananas are astringent and difficult to digest, but can be used to relieve diarrhea and colitis. Eaten ripe—when the brown speckles begin to appear—the fruit is sweet, easily digested, and soothing to the mucus lining of the stomach. (Placing bananas in a closed brown paper bag will speed the ripening process.)

VERY BERRY PUDDING

The bananas lend a rich creaminess to this puréed berry treat.

Bananas, ripe with brown speckles
Berries, fresh or frozen

In a food processor or blender, purée the bananas and berries together. Continue to add fruit until you reach a consistency you like. For a deeper color and more berry flavor, just add more berries. If using frozen berries, you don't need to refrigerate before serving. Otherwise, refrigerate for at least 1 hour. This looks great in a clear glass dish. Try making different batches, each with a single type of berry such as strawberry or blueberry, to create several different color puddings. Layer them in a parfait glass (individual size or larger) for a beautiful dessert, snack, or midafternoon meal.

Variations: Add in 1 Tbsp. of raw nut or seed butter, such as tahini, almond, or cashew, to make a richer taste.

YUMMY YAM PUDDING

Served in orange shells, this delicious, vitamin-packed treat will delight your kids as well as your most elegant dinner guests.

Serves 6.

3 large yams, baked and peeled
3 large oranges, juiced (cut oranges in half and save the orange shells)
1 ripe banana
1 oz. soft organic silken tofu
2 tsp. pure maple syrup
¾ tsp. cinnamon
⅛ tsp. nutmeg
⅛ tsp. pure vanilla extract
Fresh mint sprigs, for garnish

In a blender or food processor, purée all ingredients with enough juice to whip into a creamy, light consistency. Spoon mixture back into the orange shells. Sprinkle with cinnamon and garnish with mint. Serve warm or cold.

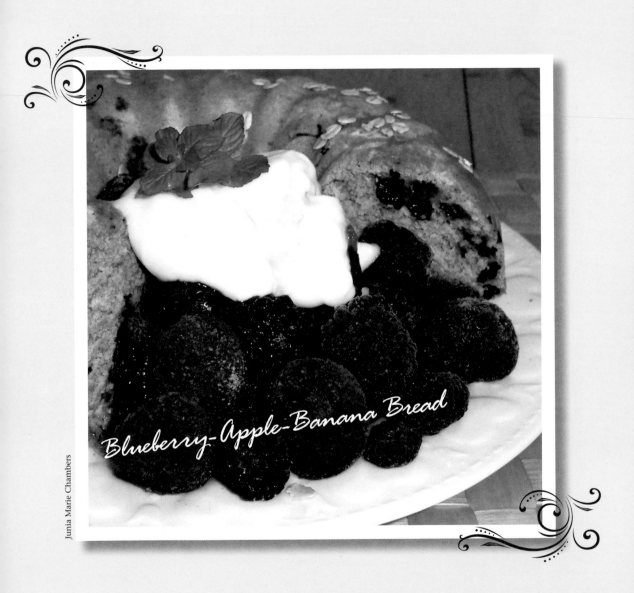

Blueberry-Apple-Banana Bread

BLUEBERRY-APPLE-BANANA BREAD

If you like banana bread, try this wonderful variation. Biting into a blueberry is like finding buried treasure. As always, this is a great thing to make when you've got overripe bananas on your hands.

Serves 5–8.

4 cups oat flour
3 ripe bananas, mashed
1 cup apple juice
1 cup frozen blueberries (or blackberries)
2½ tsp. baking powder
1 tsp. pure vanilla extract
½ tsp. cinnamon
¼ tsp. allspice
Nonstick cooking spray
Rolled oats

Preheat oven to 300° F. In a blender or food processor, blend the bananas, apple juice, and vanilla until smooth. In a large bowl, combine the flour, baking powder, cinnamon, and allspice. Add to the banana mixture in 2 batches, blending each time. Return batter to the bowl and stir in the frozen blueberries (if they thaw, the juice will run). Pour into a nonstick loaf pan that's been lightly sprayed with nonstick cooking spray. Sprinkle with a few rolled oats on top. Bake 50–60 minutes or until a knife comes out clean. Let cool before slicing and serving.

Variations: I usually make a double batch and bake it in a bundt pan. If you drizzle on an icing or berry frosting or garnish it with a variety of berries, you'll receive compliments galore.

BLUEBERRY-BONANZA SMOOTHIE

The color alone makes this one a hit with kids. Loaded with the antioxidant properties of berries and with a splash of protein from protein powder, this nutritious "shake" makes a great snack you can give to your kids with no guilt.
Serves 1–2.

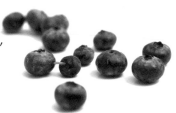

1 cup freshly squeezed organic apple or orange juice
½ cup fresh or frozen organic blueberries, strawberries, or raspberries (or a combination)
1 Tbsp. protein powder
2–3 ice cubes

Blend all ingredients in a blender or food processor until creamy smooth.
Variation: In place of the powder, use a quarter cup of raw cashews.

FYI: Blueberries

Blueberries are one of the foods highest in antioxidants. Just ½ cup a day retards aging and can even reverse failing memory; it's referred to as the "brain berry." I keep several packages of frozen organic blueberries on hand in my freezer so that I don't run out.

PURPLE GRAPE JULIUS

Another colorful and frothy juice treat kids just love.
Serves 2–3.

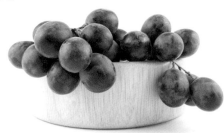

1 cup freshly squeezed purple grape juice (or bottled)
1 cup freshly squeezed orange juice (or from a carton)
½ cup frozen red or purple seedless grapes
1 Tbsp. protein powder
2–3 ice cubes

In a blender, combine all of the ingredients and blend until creamy smooth.

FYI: Grapes

Red grapes and red-grape juice have moderate antioxidant power, but purple-grape juice tops most other juices in antioxidant activity, having 4 times more than orange or tomato juice.

CREAMY-CASHEW & APPLE-CINNAMON SMOOTHIE

I always keep raw cashews in my freezer. They're a versatile nut that I use in a variety of ways.

Serves 2–3.

1½ cups apple juice
½ cup almond milk (see Chapter 2)
2 oz. organic silken tofu (or 3 oz. nondairy yogurt)
¼ cup raw cashews
2 ice cubes
Cinnamon

In a blender, combine all ingredients and blend until smooth.

FYI: Soy Milk

Milk from the soybean is similar to cow's milk, but without the cholesterol or dairy allergens. It has the same amount of protein but only ⅓ the fat, fewer calories, no cholesterol, many essential B vitamins, and 15 times as much iron. It comes in plain, vanilla, and chocolate in all natural-food stores and most supermarkets. It can be used in any dish calling for cow's milk—breakfast cereal, smoothies, casseroles, soups, pudding, quick breads, pancakes, or by the glassful as a beverage. Look for organic soy milk, or you can make it yourself, as I do, with a soy-milk machine. (See the Resources section for ordering information.) It takes only minutes, you can use organic soybeans, and it costs less than 25 cents a quart. I make a batch weekly and add pure vanilla extract when I want vanilla flavor. I also use the same machine to make delicious, fresh tofu. There are many ways to use tofu: diced on salads; grilled as steaks; for tofu burgers; or blended into dressings, smoothies, dips, and puddings.

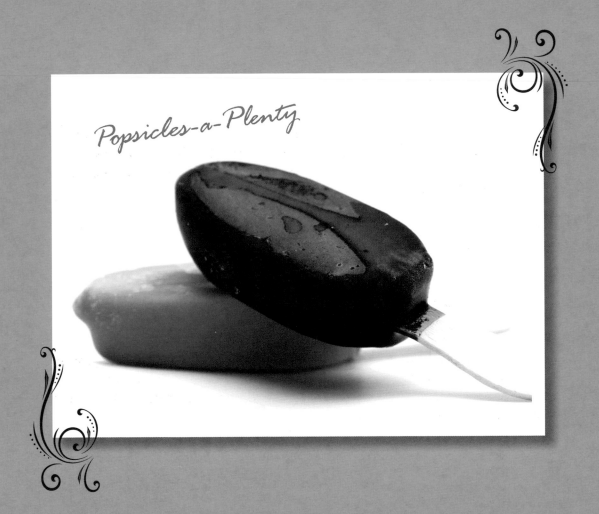

Popsicles-a-Plenty

POPSICLES-A-PLENTY

These Popsicles are a fun variation on the simple frozen-fruit treat. With no added sugar or colorings, these natural and refreshing ices are a great snack on a hot day. They'll last a month in the freezer, but I guarantee you won't have them around that long.

Popsicle molds
Fresh juice of your choice
Purified water

Fill each Popsicle mold with a combination of ½ fruit juice and ½ purified water. Fresh juice is always the best, but any natural juice will do. Freeze and enjoy.

Variations: Try adding fresh fruit, such as berries, diced pineapple, or peaches, to the juice in the Popsicle mold, and for another special treat, pour in your favorite fruit smoothie and freeze. You can also freeze in layers with different juices so that you have Rainbow Popsicles.

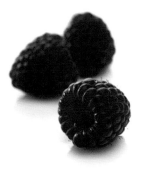

LEMON-COCONUT SHERBET

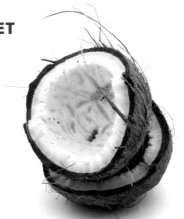

Your kids will think they're eating ice cream.
Serves 4–6.

1 coconut
⅓ cup fruit concentrate
2 tsp. fresh lemon juice
2 tsp. fresh lemon zest (from an organic lemon only)
Organic vanilla almond milk (see Chapter 2)

Open the coconut and strain the milk through a fine mesh strainer, removing any shell pieces or fiber. Set aside. Remove the coconut flesh. Juice it and save the pulp. (You can also use a young coconut and scrape out the softer coconut meat on the inside so that you don't have to juice it.)

In a bowl, combine the coconut milk, coconut juice, fruit concentrate, and pulp. Add the lemon juice and zest and enough milk to make 2 cups. Transfer the mixture to a shallow plastic or metal dish. Freeze until solid, about 4 hours. Using a knife or metal spatula, break the frozen mixture into 2- to 3-inch pieces and transfer to a food processor or blender. Purée until creamy smooth. Stop occasionally to scrape the sides. Serve immediately or store in a tightly covered plastic container in the freezer. It will keep for a month in your freezer, but I can guarantee it will be gone long before then!

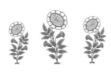

AFTERWORD
LIVING WITH COMMITMENT
& PASSION: IT'S YOUR CHOICE

". . . meditate on it day and night, so that you may be
careful to do according to all that is written; for then you
will make your way prosperous, and then you will have success."

— JOSHUA 1:8

In this Afterword, I'd like to leave you with some food for thought that I hope will inspire, motivate, and empower you to make a commitment to live your highest potential and create your best life. It has to do with how I overcame a major challenge in my life.

Many years ago, my doctor told me that because I'd fractured my back in a terrible auto accident, I'd never again be physically active and would endure chronic pain. He told me that I should get used to a life of anguish, inactivity, and difficulty; and that I'd never be able to carry anything heavier than a light purse.

I felt quite upset upon hearing this, and that accident was the impetus to change my life. I refused to believe the doctor's prognosis and turned inward, to my own Higher Power. As I began to read books and attend lectures on the power of commitment and the power of the mind to affect physical healing, I mustered up the courage and the passion to prove my doctor wrong. Within six months, I had no more pain, and the doctor said it was a miracle. My recovery proved to me that we have within ourselves everything we need to live our lives to the fullest.

Today, my health and my life have become the antithesis of that diagnosis. How did I get from the hospital bed to health, peace, and success? Well, this book, along with the other two books in the Hay House series—*Health Bliss* and *The Healing Power of NatureFoods*—provides you with the road map and all of the tools you need to experience health bliss.

Helen Keller once communicated the following: "When one door closes, another opens; but often we look so long at the closed door that we do not see the one which has opened for us." After the accident, all I could see was a closed door. I was filled with depression, self-pity, confusion, and feelings of being victimized. After a couple of weeks, I went to a favorite spot overlooking the Santa Monica Bay where I often go when I'm in need of inspiration. I had a heart-to-heart talk with myself.

On the one hand, I was convinced that life was meant to be a magnificent adventure—to be lived fully—which to me meant joyfully, passionately, healthfully, and peacefully. But the life the doctor had described wasn't like that at all. Could I accept those limitations? I knew I had a choice to make. While I didn't know exactly how I could change my physical condition, I recognized that there was a higher power within me that had the answers. So I simply made a deep decision and commitment to let go, to live from inner guidance, and to accept only vibrant, radiant health.

Of course, it hasn't always been an easy road, and I've made many mistakes. Nonetheless, I can see in retrospect that the car accident was a valuable experience, because hitting that low spot turned my life around. Someone once said, "The darker the sky, the brighter the stars." It wasn't until I made a real commitment that amazing—and what some people would call miraculous—things began to come my way. I discovered the power of belief and faith—faith meaning sometimes having to believe in things when appearances and common sense told me not to. I also discovered the power in commitment.

Here's my favorite quote on the subject. It's from *The Scottish Himalayan Expedition,* by W. H. Murray:

> Until one is committed there is hesitancy, the chance to draw back, always ineffectiveness. Concerning all acts of initiative (and creation) there is one elementary truth, the ignorance of which kills countless ideas and splendid plans: that the moment one definitely commits oneself, then Providence moves too.

All sorts of things occur to help one that would never otherwise have occurred. A whole stream of events issues from the decision, raising in one's favor all manner of unforeseen incidents and meetings and material assistance, which no man could have dreamt would have come his way. I have learned a deep respect for one of Goethe's couplets: "Whatever you can do, or dream you can, begin it. Boldness has genius, power, and magic in it."

Once I made the firm commitment to recovery, a stream of events began that assisted me in healing my condition, from finding the perfect books and tapes, to hearing certain lectures, to meeting people who told me about healing and salutary foods, visualization, and meditation (much of which sounded kind of weird to me at the time).

During the months following the accident (and to this day), I've made numerous changes in my lifestyle, behavior, thoughts, and attitude. At my six-month checkup following the accident, the doctor shook his head in bewilderment and said, "This just can't be. There is no sign of a fracture, and you seem to be in perfect health, free of pain. There must be some mistake. It's just miraculous." Perhaps it was. Yet I've since discovered that miracles are a natural part of committing to being healthy and living peacefully.

Creating Your Best Life

It doesn't matter where your level of health is at this moment. Regardless of the lifestyle you've lived until now, you can, at any moment, choose differently. You can use your past mistakes or poor choices and learn from them, but for some people, it takes hitting bottom for them to awaken to the fact that they can choose to change.

What about you? Have you made a commitment to being healthy and living peacefully? Your level of health, right this moment, is a result of the countless choices you've made regarding the foods you eat, the exercise you get, how you deal with stress, the thoughts you think, and what you believe and expect—simply how you choose to live your life.

A commitment to choose health begins with appreciating, respecting, and loving your magnificent body. One of the most important things you can learn in life is to appreciate yourself. As you open your heart to your own self-worth and to the divine essence of all humanity, you access the most powerful healer of all—the healing power of love. The human body is indeed a miracle of love's creation. The more I study the body, the more I'm amazed and in awe of how beautifully it's designed. Clearly, the physical self is fantastic and deserves reverence.

Start today and tune in more to your body. It's a remarkable feedback machine. If you listen, you'll discover that it actually talks to you. When you get a headache, for instance, it's trying to tell you something. Listen to your body's signals with health and peace as your goals. The key here is your willingness to listen and act.

We Americans have been making some poor health choices for quite some time. Just look at all of the commercials on television and advertisements in magazines: "Here's what you can do for a headache . . . constipation . . . sleepless nights . . . diarrhea . . . indigestion . . . foot odor . . . underarm odor . . ." (My gosh, take a shower!) We've come to look outside of ourselves for "solutions" to our health problems. We've become a self-medicating society because we don't really understand how beautifully robust the human body is, or how efficiently and effectively equipped we are to overcome our problems.

Choose to Make a Positive Difference

I have some astonishing news for you. It's normal to be able to go to sleep at night without taking a pill. It's normal to *not* have headaches, sinus problems, hemorrhoids, constipation, and shaky hands. It's normal to be well. We just have to "get out of our own way." By doing so and by living more from inner guidance, we can enrich the quality of life on this planet.

I love what Erich Fromm once said: "Our highest calling in life is precisely to take loving care of ourselves." In simply doing this, we can make a difference in our world. *You* make a difference. You see, our bodies are made up of trillions of cells. In order to maintain optimal health, each of these cells must operate at peak performance. When we have sick or weak cells, the healthy or stronger ones must work harder so that our body as a whole will be healthy.

Our planet is like a body, and we're all its individual cells. In other words, we're all cells in the body of humanity. We aren't separate from our fellow humans. There's no room for negative thinking, unforgiveness, bitterness toward others, or selfishness. It's our responsibility to this body that we call our planet to be healthy, happy, peaceful, loving cells that radiate only goodness, positiveness, and joy. In this way, we can help make our world harmonious.

The separation and division that has so long colored our thoughts and beliefs regarding our lives on this planet must now be examined and corrected. To create peace on Earth, we must stop dividing the world, the nations, the races, the religions, the sexes, the ages, the families, and the resources, and know that it's time to come together and live in harmony, forgiveness, and love. The awareness of our oneness must precede our thoughts and actions as a part of our belief system. It's your choice. You can choose to make a difference with the way you live your life.

In *The Hundredth Monkey,* Ken Keyes, Jr., tells of a phenomenon observed by scientists. The eating habits of macaque monkeys were studied. One monkey discovered that by washing sweet potatoes before eating them, they tasted better. She taught her mother and friends until one day a certain number (say, 99) of the monkeys knew how to wash their sweet potatoes. The next day, when the hundredth monkey learned how to wash sweet potatoes, an amazing thing happened: the rest of the colony miraculously knew how to wash their potatoes too! Not only that, but the monkeys on other islands started washing their potatoes. Keyes applies this "Hundredth Monkey" phenomenon to humanity. When more of us individually choose to make a difference with our lives—when we realize that we *do* make a difference and start acting like it—more and more of us will hop on the bandwagon until we reach the "Millionth Person" and peace spreads across the globe.

Wherever You Go, There You Are

It starts right here where we are. I believe that we can choose to change ourselves, and as we do that, the world will be different. Together, we can create a magnificent, glorious planet. I see it changing now. My vision is clear and fantastic. But it takes all of us together, committing to being healthy and peaceful, choosing to do the things that make a difference—things that support wellness, that embrace humanity, and that serve all creation. Let's all remember that we're here not to see through one another, but to see one another through.

It's simply a matter of choice. Radiant health, peace, and living your highest vision come from making a commitment and choosing to live more from inner guidance and assisting others on their journey. When you choose to live and be this way, life will take on new meaning. You'll not only understand what it means to celebrate yourself and life, you'll also enrich the quality of life on this magnificent, wondrous planet. I salute your great adventure.

"Do not be conformed to this world, but continually be transformed by the renewing of your minds so that you may be able to determine what God's will is—what is proper, pleasing, and perfect."

— Romans 12:2

RESOURCES
SOME OF SUSAN'S FAVORITE
HEALTH PRODUCTS

"As soon as you trust yourself, you will know how to live."

— JOHANN WOLFGANG VON GOETHE

Since I receive thousands of letters asking for ordering information for my favorite health-promoting products, I thought I would list them here. Included are all of the special products mentioned in this book. I've also written a description of my favorite natural-health organization, the National Health Association.

If you visit my Website, **www.SusanSmithJones.com**, and click on "Susan's Favorite Products" and "Maximize Health," you'll find that I discuss many of them in more detail. You'll also find a variety of media interviews that you can listen to for more information.

Susan's Favorite Health Products

○ **Age in Reverse:** I wouldn't be without my Body Slant or many of their other products, which I've used for more than 30 years. **www.AgeEasy .com** (888) 243-3279 (Age-Easy)

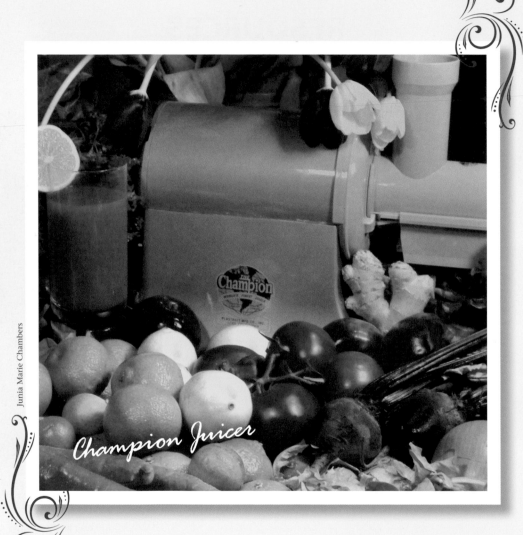

Champion Juicer

Junia Marie Chambers

- **Ancient Secrets Nasal Cleansing Pot:** www.ancient-Secrets.com/neti.cfm (877) 263-9456

- **Bernard Jensen International:** My favorite internal-cleanse products and supplements by Dr. Ellen Tart-Jensen. **www.BernardJensen.com** (760) 471-9977

- **Champion Juicer:** When it comes to power, ease of use, and versatility, nothing compares to a Champion Juicer. **www.ChampionJuicer.com** (866) 935-8423

- **E3Live:** My favorite green liquid supplement is E3Live. It's one of the best superfoods (see Chapter 10). **www.E3Live.com** (888) 800-7070 or (541) 273-2212

- **Ellen Tart-Jensen, Ph.D.:** For a free copy of her eBook *The Simplified Guide to Internal Cleansing.* **www.BernardJensen.com** (760) 471-9977

- **Eng3's device:** Powerful oxygen enhancement device (see Chapter 11). **www.Eng3corp.com** (877) 571-9206

- **Excalibur Food Dehydrator:** To dry your own fruits and vegetables at home, I recommend the Excalibur Food Dehydrator. **www.Excalibur Dehydrator.com** (800) 875-4254

- *Health Science* **magazine:** www.HealthScience.org

- **Hydro Floss:** **www.OralCareTech.com** (800) 635-3594

- **Infrared saunas:** Click on "Susan's Favorite Products" on my Website. **www.SusanSmithJones.com** add (800) 794-5355 or (303) 413-8500

- **Ionizer Plus:** This water filtration system is paramount in my health program (see Chapter 10). **www.HighTechHealth.com** (800) 794-5355 or (303) 413-8500

- **Kitchen Mill:** The best home flour grinder by far. **www.Blendtec.com** (800) 253-6383

- **Kyolic:** The most powerful (odor-free) garlic supplement. Contact them for a free sample. **www.Kyolic.com** (800) 421-2998

- **LaraBars: wwwLaraBar.com** (720) 945-1155

- **Living Harvest organic hemp products:** They supply all my favorites, such as milk, nuts, protein powder, and oil. **www.LivingHarvest.com** (866) 972-6879

- **MaxGXL, MaxWLX, and Max N•Fuze:** Three of my favorite supplements (see Chapter 11). Try them for three months and see how much better you look and feel. **www.4HealthBliss.com** (801) 316-6380

- **Miso:** My favorite misos are made by the South River Company, available at your natural-food store.

- **National Health Association:** A great source for accurate health information. **www.HealthScience.org**

- **Olbas Herbal Remedies:** I've used their natural products for more than 30 years. **www.Olbas.com** (800) 523-9971

- **Penn Herb Company, Ltd.:** I've used their herbal and other natural products, including one of my favorites—their Olbas line—for more than 30 years. I wouldn't be without their products. **www.PennHerb .com** (800) 523-9971

- **Physicians Committee for Responsible Medicine:** For all of the latest health and nutrition information. **www.NutritionMD.org**

- **Sea salt:** The purest and best is Celtic Sea Salt, from The Grain & Salt Society. **www.CelticSeaSalt.com** (800) 867-7258

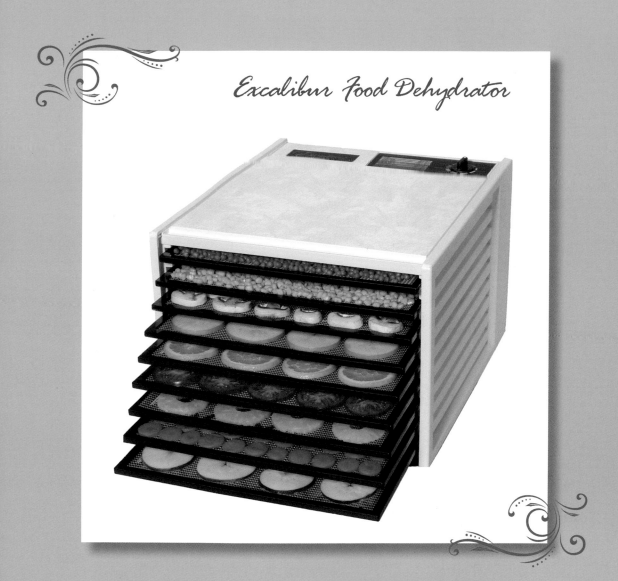

Excalibur Food Dehydrator

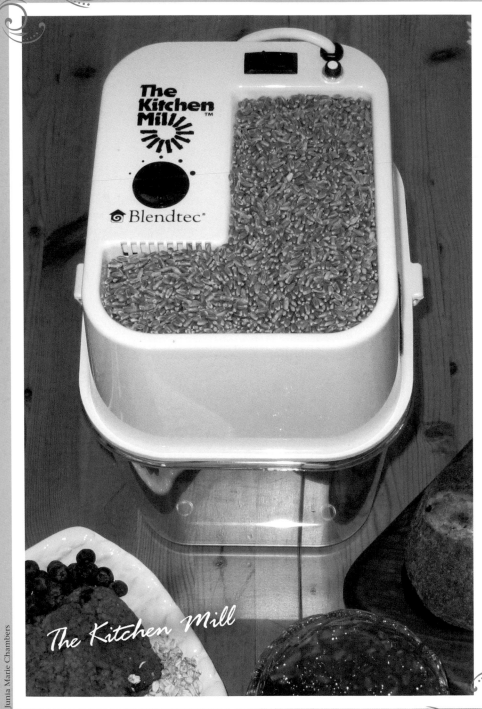

The Kitchen Mill

Junia Marie Chambers

- **Soy milk and tofu:** To make your own soy milk and tofu, I recommend the stellar SoyQuick Premier Milk Maker. **www.SoyMilkQuick. com** (888) 769-5433

- **The Grain & Salt Society: www.CelticSeaSalt.com** (800) 867-7258

- **Total Blender:** This powerful machine makes blending a joy. **www. Blendtec.com** (800) 253-6383

- **Vegetarian Cuisine:** Delicious foods prepared by gourmet Chef John B. Nowakowski, shipped frozen to your doorstep. **www.RegencyHealth Spa.com** (800) 373-7718

- **Vicki Chelf's Veggie Gobbler:** For the vegetarian or vegan Thanksgiving meal, it's a mold, complete with easy-to-follow instructions and plant-based recipes. Website: **vickisveggiegobbler.com**

- ***Well Being Journal:*** www.wellbeingjournal.com

- **Women's Healing Organization:** www.WomensHealingOrg.com

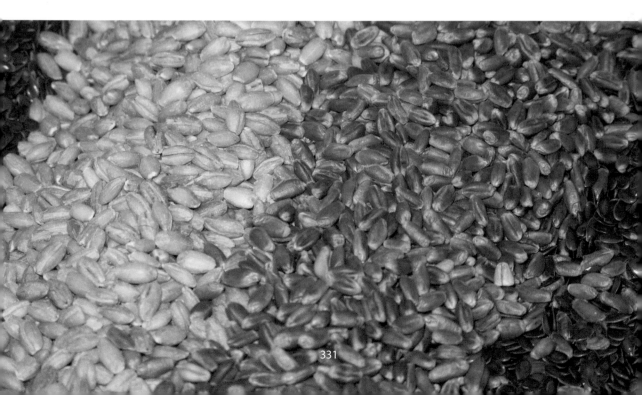

National Health Association

I encourage you to join the National Health Association (NHA). They teach you the importance of eating a plant-based, whole-foods diet; getting sufficient exercise and rest; maintaining a healthy environment; and developing psychological well-being. Members get discounts on conferences, seminars, books, and audios, and receive NHA's award-winning magazine, *Health Science.* I've been a member for 35 years, have attended dozens of conferences, purchased countless books and audio albums, written for *Health Science,* and gained a wealth of valuable knowledge that helps keep me radiantly healthy and disease free. Becoming a member of NHA is one of the best health gifts you can give yourself, and can be done quickly and easily on their Website: **www.HealthScience.org** or by calling (813) 961-6114.

JOIN SUSAN ON A EUROPEAN RETREAT

Visit: **www.SusanSmithJones.com** and learn about her special holistic health retreats on the homepage.

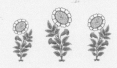

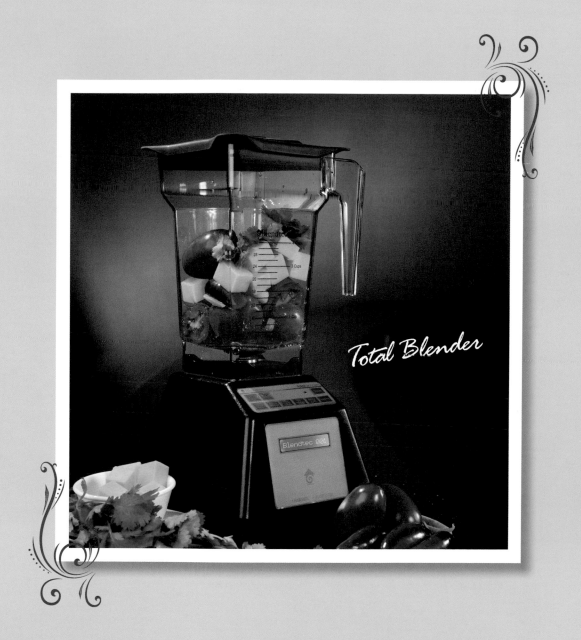

Total Blender

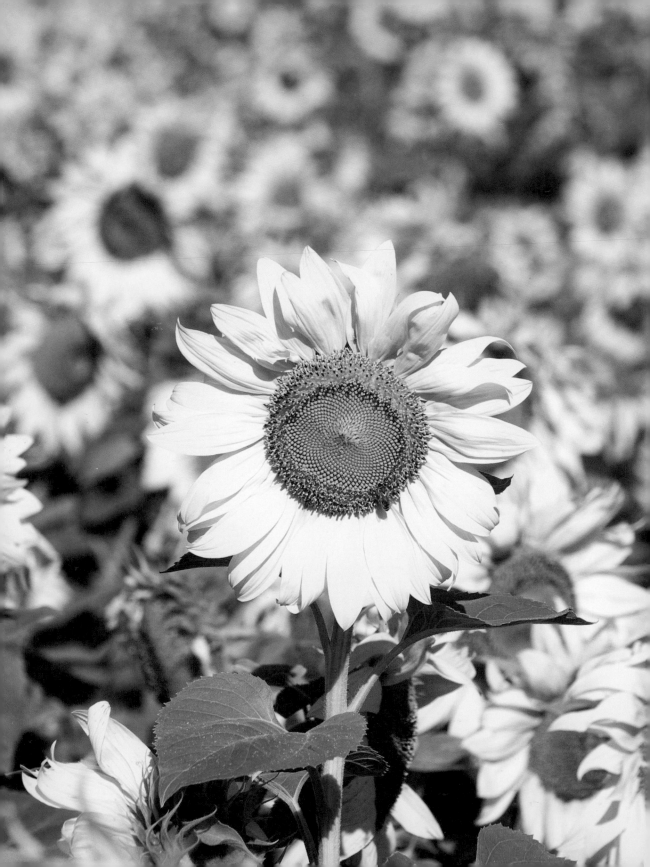

TO INSPIRE & EMPOWER

"Of course I love everyone I meet. How could I fail to? Within everyone is the spark of God. I am not concerned with racial or ethnic background or the color of one's skin; all people look to me like shining lights!"

— PEACE PILGRIM

All of the following books and audio programs by Susan Smith Jones were created individually to stand on their own—to help inspire, motivate, and empower readers and listeners. Together, however, they make the perfect *Healthy Living* gift set for you and your loved ones for any occasion.

The Healing Power of NATUREFOODS
50 Revitalizing SuperFoods & Lifestyle Choices to Promote Vibrant Health
To order: (800) 654-5126

Part of a three-book series published by Hay House (along with *Health Bliss* and *Recipes for Health Bliss*), this esteemed, empowering book demystifies nutrition facts and shows how to make appropriate food choices to decrease your risk of premature aging, heart disease, common forms of cancer, arthritis, diabetes, diminished vision, and mental functions; and to achieve permanent weight loss, reduce inflammation, and bring more vitality into your life. As a culinary instructor, private natural-food chef, and worldwide health educator extraordinaire for 30 years, Dr. Jones reveals many of her time-tested secrets on how to cleanse and detoxify your body, and offers a variety of easy-to-prepare, rejuvenating, and delicious recipes. In the face of staggering confusion about healthy nutrition and balanced living, this timeless book (and series) is a succinct guide that you'll refer to often and give away as a gift to family and friends.

HEALTH BLISS
50 Revitalizing NatureFoods & Lifestyle Choices to Promote Vibrant Health
To order: (800) 654-5126

Part of a three-book series published by Hay House (along with *The Healing Power of NATUREFOODS* and *Recipes for Health Bliss*), this acclaimed, popular book identifies 50 of the healthiest foods that heal the body and restore youthful vitality. With a Foreword by Louise L. Hay, every page of this book provides valuable information for anyone who's searching for high-level wellness and quality of life. Dr. Jones offers scrumptious, inventive, vitality-rich recipes that promise boundless pleasures for your everyday table. In addition to her reader-friendly, cutting-edge food and nutrition education, she also guides you in how to boost your metabolism, get the most from exercise, heal with delicious green smoothies, thrive from silence, experience serenity, and *look 10 years younger in less than 90 days*.

Vegetable Soup/The Fruit Bowl
To order: (800) 843-5743 • (800) 915-9355 • (941) 371-2223

This unique set of two picture books in one, created for children ages one to ten, teaches the connection between what we eat and how we feel, look, and perform. Each full-color illustration and rhyming verse has been carefully chosen to prompt interaction between the child and the reader, or between the child and the picture itself, if he or she is already reading. The entertaining text not only teaches about fresh, delicious, natural whole foods; it also helps develop math and reading skills as children take an active part. This "we are what we eat" book is the ideal way to lay the groundwork for lifelong healthy eating habits. Renowned worldwide and the winner of the Disney iParenting Media Award, this book should be recommended reading for all children; they'll thrive from it!

Be Healthy~Stay Balanced
21 Simple Choices to Create More Joy & Less Stress
To order: (800) 843-5743

Feeling physically, emotionally, and spiritually off-kilter? Lost some joy of living? Overwhelmed by life and too much stress? Wish you could look years younger and disease-proof your body? If you're in need of the perfect book to motivate you to take charge of your health, this life-changing work is for you. Dr. Jones presents an easy-to-follow program that will bring immediate, salubrious results. With a Foreword by former UCLA Basketball Coach John Wooden, you'll have at your fingertips all of the tools necessary to create a vibrantly healthy life, from a world-renowned educator who taught students, staff, and faculty at UCLA how to be healthy and fit for *30 years!*

At the end of the book, you'll find an encouraging and heartwarming CD interview with Dr. Jones that provides additional tips and tools you'll need to minimize stress and bring a sacred balance back into your body and life. It touches on all of Susan's core teachings and explores the many facets that comprise living our best lives. If you want to learn more about Susan—how she got started in holistic health, her passions, and her time-honored secrets to heal your body, look younger, and bring your highest vision to fruition—this is the perfect book/CD combination for you, your family, and your friends.

Be Healthy~Stay Balanced is one of those special books that you'll want to keep on your bedside table to uplift and inspire you before you drift off to sleep at night, as well as embrace each morning for a few minutes to start your day on a positive, healthy note. A paragon of empowerment that makes the perfect gift—this gem of a book will keep on giving for years to come.

Choose to Live Peacefully (book and audio book)
To order: (800) 843-5743 or (800) 669-0282

Many of us share a vision of world peace, a wish for harmony among all living creatures. Yet to achieve this, we must first create peace within ourselves. In this Pulitzer-nominated book, Dr. Jones offers practical guidance on how to awaken to your best self and life, including an easy-to-follow 40-day holistic body, mind, and spirit rejuvenation program. Her widespread popularity stems from her perceptive insights and positive, commonsense approach to what living healthfully and peacefully is all about. The choice is yours. Today can be the start of a peaceful new beginning in your life. In *Choose to Live Peacefully,* Dr. Jones shows you how to create an empowered presence.

You'll learn how to slow down and relax, maximize your prosperity potential, live more from trust and forgiveness, cultivate an attitude of gratitude, and live with a joyful passion. You'll attract loving, supportive relationships, learn to release fear, and live with purpose and authenticity. Dr. Jones will empower and motivate you to make your home a sanctuary, simplify your living space, and let nature nourish your soul and lift your spirit. Curl up with this book, and invite peace and love to be your constant companions.

Audio Books

Wired to Meditate (audio program)
To order: **www.SusanSmithJones.com**

This dynamic audio program explores the relationship between the mind and body and demystifies the process by providing beneficial advice on how to use meditation, deep-relaxation and breathing techniques, visualization, and positive thoughts to reduce stress and live your highest vision. Well-managed stress keeps your immune system healthy. Additionally, what you think, believe, and expect in life are also powerful influences on your well-being.

You'll learn how to use meditation, intuition, and mind power to foster success and how to live your highest vision with aplomb. Harness your inner power to heal your body, release the past, neutralize negative emotions, and bring your goals and dreams to fruition with ease and grace. Learn why it's so important to spend quality time in silence and solitude and create tranquility in the midst of chaos. Reignite your loving heart-light, surrender to your Higher Power, and receive the gifts of love and life.

EVERYDAY HEALTH—*Pure & Simple* (audio program)
Sure-Fire Tips to Heal Your Body, Restore Youthful Vitality & Renew Your Life
To order: **www.SusanSmithJones.com**

In this encouraging, heartwarming interview, Dr. Jones provides all of the tools you need to walk away from the darkness of doubt and confusion and into the light of vibrant health and peaceful living. She presents a workable scenario for living the integrated life of spirit, mind, and body. A modern Renaissance woman, Dr. Jones is a living example of the ancient wisdom, contemporary science, and 21st-century vision that she teaches. Her workshops and books are powerful and life-transforming, and this CD interview touches on her core teachings and explores the many facets that comprise living our best lives.

If you'd like to learn more about Dr. Jones—how she got started in holistic health, her passions, and her secrets to healing your body, looking younger, and bringing your highest vision to fruition—then this is the perfect audio program for you. She's interviewed by radio personality Nick Lawrence, and together they'll uplift, inspire, motivate, and empower you to create your best life. Their engaging, conversational interview brings her message to vibrant life and holds your attention from beginning to end. If you feel stuck or like you're in a "spin-cycle" lifestyle, if you've lost some of your joy in living, or if you just need some gentle, loving guidance to live in a more meaningful way, then *EveryDay Health—Pure & Simple* is perfect for you.

For more information or to order all of these titles and more, please visit: **SusanSmithJones.com.** (Visit today and learn how to receive one of Susan's popular e-books for free or to join Susan on one of her holistic health retreats in Europe, Australia, the UK, or North America.)

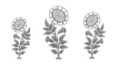

INDEX

G

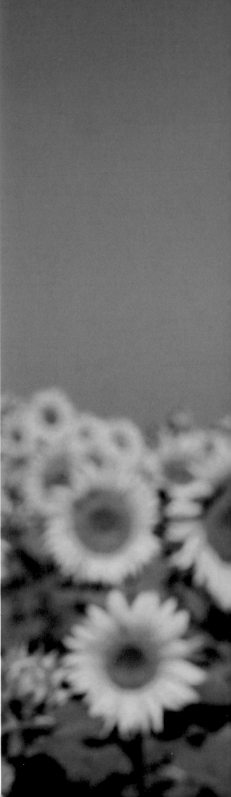

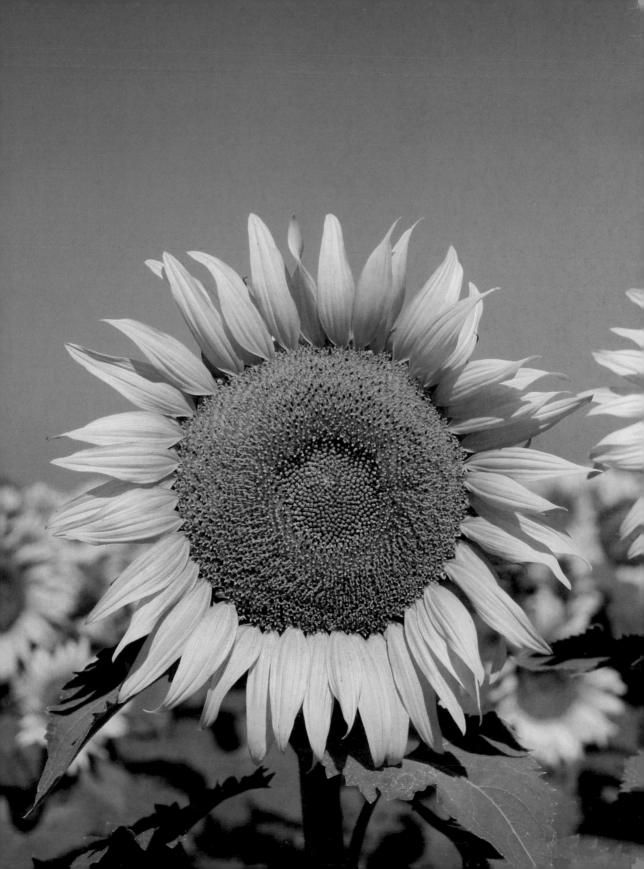

GRATITUDE

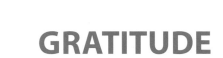

"The optimist sees opportunity in every danger; the pessimist sees danger in every opportunity. A pessimist sees the difficulty in every opportunity; an optimist sees the opportunity in every difficulty."

— Sir Winston Churchill

As I strive to live my dream with as much heart and grace as possible, there are many people who have enriched my life and assisted me in following my heart. So I'd like to take this opportunity to express my gratitude . . .

To my family—June and Reid, Jamie and Tony, Tyler and Bryce, Ad and Spark, and Jackie, for your special love, and for reminding me about what's essential, and that life is meant to be lived fully—one day at a time—with a happy heart full of gratitude.

To the most amazing publishing team in the world, comprised of more than 100 people worldwide, and most especially to Louise L. Hay, Reid Tracy, Jill Kramer, Jessica Kelley, Charles McStravick, Donna Abate, Melissa Brinkerhoff, Jami Goddess, Tricia Breidenthal, Christy Salinas, Diane Ray, Nicolette Salamanca, and Lindsay Condict, who have taught me the importance of dreaming big, and for sharing and supporting my books, vision, and heart's desire with the world.

To Junia Chambers, my dear friend, reader, photographer, and food stylist, for creating many of the photographs in this book.

To other friends who also helped bring this book to fruition, including Neal Barnard, Vicki Rae Chelf, Jean Renoux, David Knight, Victoria Moran, Nick Lawrence, Ellen Tart-Jensen, Kevin Gianni, Fléchelle Morin, Colleen and David Cox, John Robbins, Alexandra Stoddard, Ginny Swabek, Helen Guppy, Lisa Ray, Olin Idol, N.D., C.N.C, Richard Comfort, Betty Wetzel, Doncia Beath, Lori Bain, Susan and Bill Kulick, Mamiko Matsuda, Bill Betz, Jr., Karen Page, Nick Colasanti, and Rebecca Linder Hintze.

And to Christ and my celestial companions—all who nurture my spiritual side, enrich my life, and guide me along this magnificent journey with their gentle touch, wise counsel, and loving presence. Thank you for being the wind beneath my wings and showing me that with enough love, faith, trust, and patience, all challenges can be overcome, and dreams can become reality.

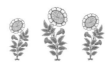

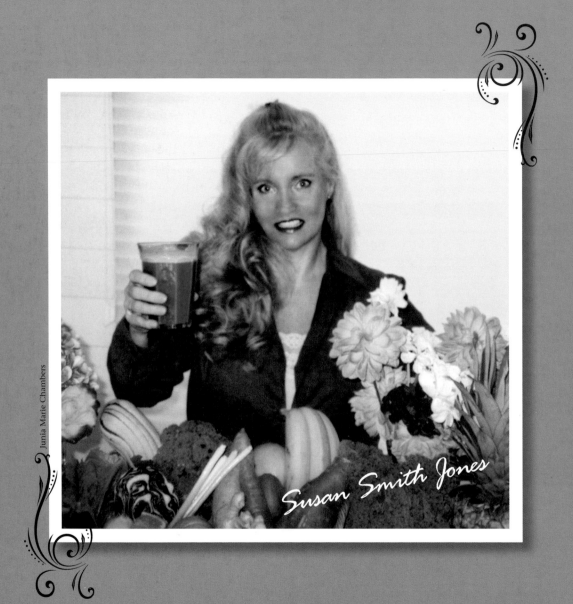

Junia Marie Chambers

Susan Smith Jones

ABOUT SUSAN SMITH JONES

"The future belongs to those who believe in the beauty of their dreams."

— Eleanor Roosevelt

For a woman with three of America's most ordinary names, **Susan Smith Jones, Ph.D.,** has certainly made extraordinary contributions in the fields of holistic health and fitness, anti-aging, optimal nutrition, and balanced living. For starters, she taught students, staff, and faculty at UCLA how to be healthy and fit for *30 years!* As a renowned motivational speaker, Susan travels internationally as a frequent radio/TV talk-show guest, keynote speaker, and holistic-lifestyle coach. She's also the author of more than 500 magazine articles and 20 books and audio programs. Some of her most popular titles include *Health Bliss; Be Healthy~Stay Balanced; Wired to Meditate; The Healing Power of NatureFoods; Healthy, Happy & Radiant . . . at Any Age; Choose to Live Fully; Choose to Live Peacefully; Renew Your Life; Simplify • Detoxify • Meditate; EveryDay Health—Pure & Simple;* and *Vegetable Soup/The Fruit Bowl* (a nutrition book for children ages one to ten).

Susan is in a unique position to testify on the efficacy of her basic message that health is the result of choice. When her back was fractured in an automobile accident, her physician told her that she'd never be able to carry anything heavier than "a small purse." Susan chose not to accept this verdict. Within six months, her pain was gone and there was no evidence of the fracture. Soon, she fully regained her health and active lifestyle. Susan attributes her healing to her whole-foods diet and the power of Spirit, faith, and determination, which led to a deep commitment to expressing her highest potential. Since that time, she has been continually active in spreading the message that anyone can choose radiant health and rejuvenation. Her inspiring message and innovative techniques for achieving total health in body, mind, and spirit have won her a grateful and enthusiastic following and have put her in constant demand internationally as a health-and-fitness consultant and educator. A gifted teacher, Susan brings together modern research and ageless wisdom in all of her work. She resides in both West Los Angeles and Oregon.

To learn more about Susan and her work, to read some of her interviews and articles, or to book her to give a motivational talk on a variety of holistic-health topics, visit: **www.SusanSmithJones.com**. If you'd like to hear two radio interviews with Susan, visit: **weeu.com/mp3/jones7108.mp3** and **weeu.com/mp3/smithjones112108.mp3**.

"There is nothing like a dream to create the future."

— Victor Hugo

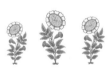

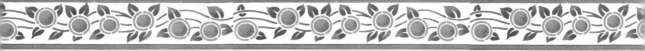

"We must learn to live together as brothers or perish as fools."

— MARTIN LUTHER KING, JR.

*"If you look at what you have in life, you'll always have more.
If you look at what you don't have, you'll never have enough."*

— OPRAH WINFREY

*"Perseverance is more prevailing than violence; and
many things that cannot be overcome when they are
together, yield themselves up when taken little by little."*

— PLUTARCH

*"Character isn't inherited. One builds it daily by the way
one thinks and acts, thought by thought, action by action."*

— HELEN GAHAGAN DOUGLAS

*"The opposite of love is not hate, it's indifference.
The opposite of faith is not heresy, it's indifference.
The opposite of life is not death, it's indifference."*

— ELIE WIESEL

"When a wise man points at the moon, the imbecile examines the finger."

— BUDDHA

"Wisdom is avoiding all thoughts that weaken you."

— LOUISE L. HAY

*"To act magnanimously, to maintain high standards,
to be honorable, requires commitment to yourself. Make it."*

— ALEXANDRA STODDARD

*"If I've learned one thing in life, it's:
Stand for something or you'll fall for anything."*

— AS QUOTED BY BONNIE HUNT

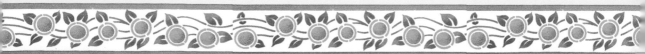

Hay House Titles of Related Interest

YOU CAN HEAL YOUR LIFE, the movie, starring Louise L. Hay & Friends
(available as a 1-DVD program and an expanded 2-DVD set)
Watch the trailer at: www.LouiseHayMovie.com

THE SHIFT, the movie,
starring Dr. Wayne W. Dyer
(available as a 1-DVD program and an expanded 2-DVD set)
Watch the trailer at: **www.DyerMovie.com**

The Answer Is Simple . . . *Love Yourself, Live Your Spirit!* by Sonia Choquette

The Art of Extreme Self-Care: *Transform Your Life One Month at a Time,*
by Cheryl Richardson

The Body Knows . . . How to Stay Young: *Healthy-Aging Secrets
from a Medical Intuitive,* by Caroline Sutherland

The Natural Nutrition No-Cook Book: *Delicious Food for YOU and Your PETS!*
by Kymythy R. Schultze

Vegetarian Meals for People-on-the-Go: *101 Quick & Easy Recipes,*
by Vimala Rodgers

Wheat-Free, Worry-Free: *The Art of Happy, Healthy, Gluten-Free Living,*
by Danna Korn

All of the above are available at your local bookstore,
or may be ordered by contacting Hay House (see last page).

We hope you enjoyed this Hay House Lifestyles book. If you'd like
to receive a free catalog featuring additional Hay House books and products,
or if you'd like information about the Hay Foundation, please contact:

Hay House, Inc.
P.O. Box 5100
Carlsbad, CA 92018-5100

(760) 431-7695 or (800) 654-5126
(760) 431-6948 (fax) or (800) 650-5115 (fax)
www.hayhouse.com® • www.hayfoundation.org

Published and distributed in Australia by: Hay House Australia Pty. Ltd.,
18/36 Ralph St., Alexandria NSW 2015 • *Phone:* 612-9669-4299
Fax: 612-9669-4144 • www.hayhouse.com.au

Published and distributed in the United Kingdom by: Hay House UK, Ltd.,
292B Kensal Rd., London W10 5BE • *Phone:* 44-20-8962-1230
Fax: 44-20-8962-1239 • www.hayhouse.co.uk

Published and distributed in the Republic of South Africa by:
Hay House SA (Pty), Ltd., P.O. Box 990, Witkoppen 2068
Phone/Fax: 27-11-467-8904 • orders@psdprom.co.za • www.hayhouse.co.za

Published in India by: Hay House Publishers India, Muskaan Complex,
Plot No. 3, B-2, Vasant Kunj, New Delhi 110 070 • *Phone:* 91-11-4176-1620
Fax: 91-11-4176-1630 • www.hayhouse.co.in

Distributed in Canada by: Raincoast, 9050 Shaughnessy St., Vancouver, B.C.
V6P 6E5 • *Phone:* (604) 323-7100 • *Fax:* (604) 323-2600 • www.raincoast.com

Tune in to **HayHouseRadio.com**® for the best in inspirational
talk radio featuring top Hay House authors! And, sign up via the
Hay House USA Website to receive the Hay House online newsletter
and stay informed about what's going on with your favorite authors.
You'll receive bimonthly announcements about Discounts and Offers,
Special Events, Product Highlights, Free Excerpts, Giveaways, and more!
www.hayhouse.com®